Scaling up health service delivery:

from pilot innovations to policies and programmes

Edited by Ruth Simmons, Peter Fajans, and Laura Ghiron

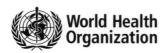 World Health Organization

EXPAND**NET**

WHO Library Cataloguing-in-Publication Data

Scaling up health service delivery: from pilot innovations to policies and programmes/edited by Ruth Simmons, Peter Fajans, and Laura Ghiron.

1.Delivery of health care. 2.Health services administration. 3.Family planning services. 4.Reproductive health services - organization and administration. I.Simmons, Ruth. II.Fajans, Peter. III.Ghiron, Laura.

ISBN 978 92 4 156351 2 (NLM classification: WA 550)

Scaling up health service delivery: from pilot innovations to policies and programmes

Printed in Switzerland

Contents

Preface

The term "scaling up" is widely used these days in many different settings – in discussions about the needed responses to the HIV/AIDS crisis, in efforts to provide for the sexual and reproductive health needs of adolescents or in programmes to bring the benefits of health technologies and interventions to the disadvantaged. In the field of development, professionals talk about scaling up initiatives to eradicate poverty, address gender inequities and preserve the world's limited natural resources. In spite of, or perhaps because of, the wide use of the term, there is no consensus on the concept's precise definition and meaning among the different people who use it. However, the sense of urgency with which the topic is raised stems from a shared concern: governments, nongovernmental organizations, and technical assistance and research institutions increasingly acknowledge that the goals of health for all, poverty eradication, sustainable development and social equity are not being reached at an acceptable pace. Current efforts need to be multiplied several times over to meet the health and development challenges facing the world at the beginning of the 21st century. This strongly felt need is aptly captured by the term "scaling up".

This book which I have the pleasure of introducing to you considers the topic of scaling up from a particular vantage point. The focus here is on ways to increase the impact of health service innovations that have been tested in pilot or experimental projects so as to benefit more people and to foster policy and programme development on a lasting, sustainable basis. The book addresses a major failure in the global health and development field: namely, the failure to expand the many successful small-scale pilot or demonstration projects that have been organized around the world so as to benefit larger populations than those initially served. It presents a conceptual framework for thinking about scaling up as well as case-studies from Africa, Asia and Latin America where the potential for expansion was a concern from the very inception of pilot or experimental projects. The case-studies discuss family planning and related reproductive health service interventions as well as other innovations in primary health care. The value of the book, however, is not limited to the specific health areas covered in the case-studies. Anyone who seeks to use the lessons of small-scale initiatives as a means of fostering larger-scale policy and programme development can learn much from it.

The case-studies presented here share a series of common values. They emphasize the imperative to build capacity within public sector institutions to meet the health needs of the disadvantaged. They highlight the necessity of building a strong sense of both local and national ownership in the identification of priority health needs, the development and testing of local solutions, and the formulation of context-specific strategies for expanding small-scale successes. They also demonstrate that, if scaling up is taken into account from the design phase of an innovation, more people eventually will benefit.

The book builds upon nearly 15 years of experience with the development and testing, in more than 25 countries around the world, of the Strategic Approach to Strengthening Reproductive Health Policies and Programmes. The Strategic Approach has dedicated deliberate attention to scaling up from its inception in the early 1990s. The Department of Reproductive Health and Research of the World Health Organization is now pleased to present this book to the many constituencies in our field who are driven by the sense of urgency that more needs to be done to expand access to high-quality sexual and reproductive health services. I hope that readers will benefit from the lessons presented and will in turn be inspired to put new insights into action.

Paul F.A. Van Look, MD PhD FRCOG
Director
Department of Reproductive Health and Research
World Health Organization, Geneva
Switzerland

Acknowledgements

Writing about scaling up was a challenging experience for all the authors who contributed to this publication. We deeply appreciate their willingness to engage with the complex subject matter and to participate in the multiple revisions necessary to highlight the key insights that emerged from their experiences. None of this would have been possible without the opportunity to meet in the serene and peaceful environment of the Rockefeller Foundation's Bellagio Study and Conference Center, for which we and all the authors are extremely grateful. The two team residencies and the conference held there gave participants the opportunity to take time out from their busy schedules to reflect, to exchange ideas, and to write, review and rewrite their contributions to this book. The beauty and comfort of the Bellagio Center and above all the gracious and supportive hospitality of Gianna Celli and the staff made a special contribution to our ability to be productive. We are also appreciative of the financial support received from the Bill and Melinda Gates Foundation, the MacArthur Foundation, the World Health Organization and the University of Michigan. Many individuals have reviewed the chapters and assisted with multiple revisions. Marge Berer's insightful review of the papers challenged us to push the presentation and analysis to the next level; Alexis Ntabona's supportive guidance in the rewriting assured us that we were on the right path, and Max Heirich's unfaltering willingness to help with a broad range of tasks sustained us throughout. We also thank Amanda Abbott and Joanna Drescher for their excellent research assistance.

Ruth Simmons
School of Public Health, University of Michigan
Ann Arbor, Michigan, USA

Peter Fajans
Department of Reproductive Health and Research
World Health Organization, Geneva
Switzerland

Laura Ghiron
School of Public Health, University of Michigan
Ann Arbor, Michigan, USA

Abbreviations

AIDS	Acquired immunodeficiency syndrome
CEMICAMP	Center for Mother and Child Research of Campinas (Brazil)
CHPS	Community-based Health Planning and Services (Ghana)
CPIRC	China Population and Information Research Center (now China Population and Development Research Center)
DMPA	Depot-medroxyprogesterone acetate
ECC	Expanding Contraceptive Choice programme (Zambia)
GTZ	Gesellschaft für Technische Zusammenarbeit (German Agency for Technical Cooperation)
HIV	Human immunodeficiency virus
ICDDR,B	International Centre for Diarrhoeal Disease Research, Bangladesh (now Centre for Health and Population Research)
ICPD	International Conference on Population and Development
IEC	Information, education and communication
IIRR	Institute for International Rural Reconstruction
IPPF	International Planned Parenthood Federation
IUD	Intrauterine device
NCPFP	National Committee of Population and Family Planning (Viet Nam)
NPFPC	National Population and Family Planning Commission (China)
NGO	Nongovernmental organization
PPMED	Policy Planning, Monitoring and Evaluation Division (Ghana)
PRP	Pilots to Regional Programmes (Zambia)
RTI	Reproductive tract infection
SFPC	State Family Planning Commission (China)
SUS	Sistema Único de Saúde (Unified Health System, Brazil)
STI	Sexually transmitted infection
UNAIDS	Joint United Nations Programme on HIV/AIDS
UNFPA	United Nations Population Fund

UNICEF	United Nations Children's Fund
USAID	United States Agency for International Development
VWU	Viet Nam Women's Union
WHO	World Health Organization

Introduction

In the past decade, a global movement has emerged to promote equitable access to high-quality reproductive health services. Its key aims have been to broaden the range of services available, to remove barriers to the utilization of care, and to ensure that providers are technically competent and respect human dignity and rights. A key strategy for reaching these goals has been to organize small-scale projects designed to test service interventions that have the potential for achieving these outcomes *(1, 2)*. Thus, hundreds of reproductive health pilot or experimental projects have been launched in developing countries, most of which have been able to demonstrate impressive success. The overall impact of such projects has been limited, however, as their influence has tended to remain confined to the original target areas, representing a failure to meet the needs of the underserved on the scale that is required *(3, 4)*.

The community of reproductive health advocates, programme managers and researchers has given little systematic attention to how the benefits achieved in successful pilot or experimental projects can be expanded to serve more people, more quickly and more equitably. The presumption has been that good ideas will spread of their own accord. While spontaneous diffusion of service innovations can occur, scaling up typically requires active sponsorship and concerted efforts from multiple stakeholders. Inadequate knowledge of the factors that lead to successful scale-up is an important reason why service innovations have had limited impact. There is little conceptual development in the health field that can guide our thinking.[1] Although relevant literature exists, it is scattered across a range of development areas and is often directed at the content of interventions rather than at the process of scaling up or determinants of its success. This book seeks to fill these gaps by:

- drawing attention to insights from relevant literature found in a variety of fields and disciplines;
- presenting a conceptual framework for thinking about the process of scaling up experimental or pilot projects;
- critically examining experience with scaling up health service pilot or experimental projects from Africa, Asia and Latin America through the use of case-studies;
- identifying practical lessons derived from the case-studies, as well as future directions for research.

---

[1] For exceptions see DeJong (5) and Cooley and Kohl. (6).

Scaling up is defined here as efforts to increase the impact of innovations successfully tested in pilot or experimental projects so as to benefit more people and to foster policy and programme development on a lasting basis. We are referring to innovations that have been tested within the country context in which they will be scaled up. This definition is more specific than when the term is used in a general sense to mean broadening the use and impact of existing or new practices, for example, "to efficiently increase the socioeconomic impact from a small to a large scale of coverage" (7). Innovation refers to a health service practice or a package of practices that are new or perceived as new in a particular programme context. This book deals with scaling up in public sector health service delivery systems. Case-studies presented cover the expansion of evidence-based contraceptive service and related reproductive health innovations in public sector programmes in Bangladesh, Bolivia, Brazil, Chile, China, Ghana, Viet Nam and Zambia. The main focus is on improving access and quality of care within a philosophy that accents human dignity and rights in reproductive health service delivery. In Ghana, service innovations involved primary health care, including family planning. In each setting a multifaceted approach to service improvement was adopted, incorporating a philosophy of reproductive health and rights and covering the organization of services, introduction of new technologies, strengthening of providers' competence, and managerial processes.

Until recently the term scaling up was used rarely in the health literature. In the last few years, however, it has become more prominent as reflected in titles such as *Scaling up, scaling down: overcoming malnutrition in developing countries (8), Getting to scale in young adults reproductive health programs (9)*, or *Making an impact in HIV and AIDS: NGO experiences of scaling up (5)*. A major focus has been on providing universal access to antiretroviral therapy for HIV-positive individuals, through efforts by the World Health Organization (WHO), the Global Fund to Fight AIDS, Tuberculosis and Malaria, and the Joint United Nations Programme on HIV/AIDS (UNAIDS). Calls to scale up result from a sense of urgency that not enough is being accomplished to meet pressing health and development needs. More must be done so that everyone reaps the benefits of medical science and health technologies, agricultural innovations, natural resource management, education and nutrition.

In some respects, the concern with scaling up is both old and new. It is related to areas of investigation that have a long history of attention under such rubrics as technology transfer, research or knowledge utilization, diffusion of innovation, research dissemination, putting research into practice and bridging the research–policy gap (10–14).

Each of these topics is associated with an extensive literature, which touches upon many of the themes that are central to the scaling up of pilot projects. Growing recognition in most of these fields is that "data seldom speak for themselves" *(15)* and that research-based recommendations are rarely sufficient to change practice *(16)*. Getting research results into wide use requires deliberate activities to push new insights into the policy process and to facilitate the adoption of new ideas and practices by managers, providers and other stakeholders. Moreover, utilization of new knowledge and practices does not occur through a logically ordered sequence of stages from problem identification and research to policy formulation and programme influence. Instead, if research is to be influential, more interactive, iterative and process-oriented approaches are needed *(17, 18)*.

Seven key themes emerged from reviews of relevant literature, analyses and discussions at three meetings held at the Rockefeller Foundation's Bellagio Study and Conference Center, and the experience of the participants with scaling up reproductive health and other primary health-care projects around the world. This book highlights the key themes identified for scaling up interventions, as follows:

- an explicit normative rationale;
- the multidimensional character of the scaling-up process;
- continuing participation by stakeholders;
- innovations adapted to local conditions;
- going to scale as a learning process;
- designing innovations with scaling up in mind;
- the need for research on scaling up.

First and foremost among these themes is the articulation of an explicit normative rationale. Powerful ethical principles concerning human dignity and human rights justify global attention to the reproductive health agenda and make scaling up imperative. Thus an important workshop organized in Manila by the Institute for International Rural Reconstruction (IIRR) emphasized a people-centred vision of health and development, with attention to issues of quality and quantity, equity and sustainability *(19, 20)*. The Manila meeting defined the objective of scaling up as providing "more quality benefits to more people over a wider geographical area more quickly, more equitably and more lastingly" *(19)*. The cases presented here share these broad objectives. Additionally, they highlight a commitment to the principles of reproductive choice and rights.

The second key theme draws attention to the fact that scaling up is multidimensional, involving not only technology transfer and the dissemination of information. It is a more complex social, political and institutional process than was recognized earlier. Occurring within a web of interacting forces, going to scale must engage multiple actors, interest groups and organizations, while taking account of the larger socioeconomic, political, cultural and institutional contexts within which it takes place. Dealing with these varied environments is not a neutral process but often touches upon complex political relationships that can provide major challenges as one seeks to enhance organizational capacity and institution-building (7, 19).

Third, a commitment to participation involving a broad range of stakeholders is considered fundamental, and this commitment must exist from the stage of developing an innovation, all the way through the process of scaling up. Involvement of local people in decision-making, and responsiveness to community interests, are essential elements of participatory approaches. At the same time, the book emphasizes that attaining true participation and the expected benefits of community empowerment is not easy. Stakeholder groups are likely to approach the scaling-up task from a variety of perspectives, needs and interests, and they interact with each other in the context of unequal power relationships.

Fourth, adaptation of innovations to ensure a good fit with local needs and circumstances is repeatedly highlighted. The need for adaptation is still insufficiently appreciated in practice. The expectation that easily replicable innovations can be discovered and readily disseminated continues to distort understandings of how scaling up can be accomplished.

Fifth, scaling up is viewed as a learning process that involves building local capacities for innovation, and undertaking the needed adaptation of tested innovations to local settings. This idea was succinctly articulated in the IIRR seminar report, which states that going to scale implies more than replication. It also refers to the dissemination or expansion of "options, knowledge, processes and technologies such that people build capacities to make better decisions and/or influence decision-making authorities" (19, p. 21). Ensuring that learning and capacity building do in fact take place typically involves new and creative educational or training efforts, especially in situations where the desired change is extensive.

Reinforcing recent views from the literature on research utilization, the sixth theme insists on a new relationship between research and its broader dissemination and utilization. Previously, researchers often designed and tested innovations and then passed on the scaling-up task to others. In contrast, the present authors argue that pilot or demonstration projects should be undertaken with the implications of scaling up in mind, rather than turning to this task as an afterthought once research is completed. Policy-makers and programme managers as well as other users of research should be involved from the beginning, and the financial and organizational requirements of scaling up must be considered from the outset. Thus we use the term scaling up in both a broad and a narrow sense: in the broadest sense it refers to the entire process that begins with the design and testing of an innovation and then proceeds to its expansion to other areas or groups of people; in the narrow, more conventional sense it does not include the design and testing of the innovation but covers only the process of expansion or replication.

The final theme of the book highlights that the process and outcomes of scaling up should be the focus of research, so that the determinants of successful scaling up can be better understood and recorded for later reference by other initiatives seeking to amplify their impact. This is not usually the case. Scaling up tends to be considered a part of routine programme operations not requiring systematic research and evaluation. This is one of the reasons for the failure to achieve large impact and explains why scaling up must be the subject of research as well.

The chapters of this book were first presented as papers at a 2003 conference, the second of three Bellagio meetings entitled "From pilot projects to policies and programmes". The conference, jointly organized by the University of Michigan and the World Health Organization (WHO), grew out of more than a decade of work on the Strategic Approach to Strengthening Reproductive Health Policies and Programmes. The Strategic Approach is a methodology that countries can use to identify and prioritize their needs with regard to reproductive health technologies and services; test appropriate interventions to address these priority needs; and then scale up successful interventions to a regional or national level. It involves both the testing and expansion of health service innovations (21–24).

The three stages of the Strategic Approach – strategic assessment, action research and scaling up – are geared towards decision-making based on an understanding of the service context and its capabilities; client needs, perspectives and rights; and available technological and service delivery options. The first stage consists of an interdisciplinary and participatory strategic assessment designed to identify critical service interventions, policy recommendations and research needs that are likely to improve access, availability and the quality of health services. Pilot projects and related service delivery research are then undertaken to test recommendations from the assessment. The third stage uses the results of the assessment and action research to encourage policy planning and programmatic action. The Strategic Approach has been implemented in 25 countries in Africa, Asia, central and eastern Europe, Latin America and the Middle East.

When the first country projects working with this methodology reached the stage of scaling up, the group of partners working with WHO on the development and implementation of the Strategic Approach realized the need to learn more about the determinants of successful scaling up. This led to extensive literature reviews, development of a conceptual framework, and the three Bellagio meetings. The first meeting, in 2001, allowed a retrospective review of experiences with implementing the Strategic Approach from the perspective of scaling up. Participants discussed the following three central questions: How would the strategic assessment have been conducted differently if scaling up had been a concern, and had been better understood, from the outset? What has been learned about conducting pilot or demonstration research in ways that enhance the potential for widespread impact of the results? What facilitates and what hinders the scaling up of successful pilot or experimental projects?

The participants produced a series of key questions requiring further examination and agreed that they should be explored in the preparation of papers about specific country experiences. The points to be examined focused on what has been learned about:

- maintaining and institutionalizing the basic values and philosophies of human rights and gender perspectives in the process of expanding the impact of pilot and experimental projects;
- building and maintaining participatory processes and ownership while taking projects to scale;
- ensuring that political, policy, legal and institutional scaling up take place;
- developing the human resources and appropriate training and educational strategies for achieving quality of care and sustainable scale-up;
- building and sustaining the resource team's capacity to give technical assistance throughout the process of expansion;
- designing pilot, demonstration or experimental projects to maximize and ensure sustainable scale-up;
- measuring success and monitoring and evaluating the process to facilitate learning;

- sustaining scaling up in decentralized, bureaucratic, resource-constrained and changing health-care systems undergoing health sector reform.

Subsequent to the first meeting at the Bellagio Study and Conference Center, the 2003 conference was organized with the objectives of further clarifying a conceptual framework and methodologies for advancing the science and practice of scaling up; contributing to the available empirical evidence through the presentation of country case-studies; and informing the field of practice. Conference participants included policy-makers, programme managers, trainers and applied researchers from countries that had implemented the Strategic Approach, as well as from two other major scaling-up programmes: the Chinese Quality-of-Care Project and the Ghana Community-based Health Planning and Services initiative. In addition, the conference was attended by professionals with expertise in reproductive health policy, programming and implementation, and in health sector reform. During the meeting, conference participants founded a global network, called ExpandNet, dedicated to enhancing scientific understanding of scaling up and its practical applications. The chapters in this book were further elaborated at the final team residency in Bellagio in 2004.

Chapter 1 provides a conceptual framework for thinking about the scaling-up process within a systems context. The framework is informed by the literature of several disciplines and seeks to promote an interdisciplinary perspective on the topic. It has been strongly influenced by discussions among Strategic Approach partners as they implemented a variety of projects over the years. Insights from the policy, organization and social sciences, as well as from the family planning, health and development fields, are utilized to characterize the complex system within which scaling up takes place and to articulate the strategic choices that must be made as successful pilot and experimental projects are expanded.

Then case-studies are presented from Asia, Africa and Latin America. Chapter 2 describes the process of scaling up the introduction of the injectable contraceptive depot-medroxyprogesterone acetate (DMPA) while improving quality of care for all contraceptive methods in Viet Nam's national family planning programme. This initiative first developed a comprehensive set of materials and tools to support strengthening quality of care. These were tested in demonstration sites prior to being used to develop broader capacity to implement reproductive choice within a centralized, bureaucratic and demographically focused programme environment. This account focuses on the challenges involved in maintaining quality as interventions are rapidly scaled up to broad programme implementation.

Chapter 3 discusses the quality of care reform in China, which seeks to focus the family planning programme on client needs, informed choice of contraceptives, and better quality services. Partly inspired by the 1994 International Conference on Population and Development (ICPD) and the 1995 Beijing Women's Conference, the reform began as a pilot project among six counties and has now become a blueprint for reorienting the national programme. The China case-study reviews the process by which this innovative experiment was scaled up into a national reform effort and the key lessons learned about scaling up sensitive but needed innovations in a complex political environment.

The discussion in Chapter 4 moves to Zambia, reporting on a project that initially field-tested a package of activities to support service delivery in three rural health districts of the Copperbelt Province. The project strengthened contraceptive choice, developed referral systems for methods not available on site, and applied innovative approaches to provider training. These innovations were then scaled up to the entire Copperbelt in an approach that promoted a common set of quality standards while maintaining flexibility in the implementation of activities based on local needs and conditions.

The next two chapters are about the Community-based Health Planning and Services (CHPS) initiative in Ghana, which has successfully replicated within the national health programme the experimental service delivery innovations developed and tested by the Navrongo Health Research Centre in northern Ghana. Using locally available resources, the initiative has demonstrated the feasibility of reorienting primary health care from clinics to communities by mobilizing traditional social institutions to foster volunteerism, community support and decentralized planning.

Chapter 5 highlights the importance of scaling-up strategies that phase in change incrementally, emphasize learning processes, engage in decentralized planning and adapt strategies to local circumstances and need.

Chapter 6 compares the Ghana CHPS initiative with the scaling up in Bangladesh of health service innovations first tested in the Matlab Maternal Child Health and Family Planning Project. The account shows that large-scale programme development was achieved not because the scaling-up strategies were alike, but because similar research approaches informed their strategies and allowed them to adapt to contrasting societal and institutional contexts.

The two final chapters discuss scaling up related to the Reprolatina Project in Latin America. This project sought to expand service innovations and participatory approaches pioneered in connection with the Strategic Approach in Brazil to other municipalities in that country and to Bolivia and Chile. Chapter 7 focuses on Brazil, addressing the question of what has been learned about sustainable scaling up in resource-constrained, decentralized public sector settings, while Chapter 8 describes an innovative training and educational methodology applied in Bolivia, Brazil and Chile as the means of scaling up technical and managerial improvements in the public sector.

The case-studies in this book address primarily contraceptive and related reproductive health services. The theoretical framework and many of the insights derived from these studies are not limited to reproductive health, however, but can be applied to other areas of health and development. The determinants of success often apply across sectors because the policy, planning, organizational, management, and monitoring tasks are generic to all scaling-up initiatives. We hope that the approaches and findings discussed here are of value to programme managers and researchers who seek to enhance the impact of pilot and experimental projects so as to benefit more people and foster policy and programme development on a lasting basis.

References

1. Jowell R. *Trying it out – the role of 'pilots' in policy-making: report of a review of government pilots.* Edinburgh, National Centre for Social Research, 2003.

2. Partners for Health Reformplus. *The role of pilot programs – approaches to health systems strengthening.* Bethesda, MD, Abt Associates Inc., 2004.

3. Koenig MA, Whittaker M. Increasing the application of operations research findings in public sector family planning programs: lessons from the ICDDR,B Extension Project. In: Seidman M, Horn MC, eds. *Operations research: helping family planning programs work better.* New York, Wiley-Liss Inc., 1991:451–460.

4. Phillips JF, Simmons R, Simmons G. The institutionalization of operations research. In: Seidman M, Horn MC, eds. *Operations research: helping family planning programs work better.* New York, Wiley-Liss Inc., 1991:503–530.

5. DeJong J. *Making an impact in HIV and AIDS: NGO experiences of scaling up.* London, Intermediate Technology Development Group Publishing, 2003.

6. Cooley L, Kohl R. *Scaling up – from vision to large-scale change: A management framework for practitioners.* Washington, DC, Management Services International, 2005. (http://www.msiworldwide.com/documents/ScalingUp.pdf, accessed 6 April 2006).

7. *Scaling up the impact of good practices in rural development: a working paper to support the implementation of the World Bank's rural development strategy.* Washington, DC, The World Bank, Agriculture and Rural Development Department, 2003 (Report No. 26031).

8. Marchione TJ, ed. *Scaling up, scaling down: overcoming malnutrition in developing countries.* Amsterdam, Gordon Breach Publishers, 1999.

9. Smith J, Colvin C. *Getting to scale in young adults' reproductive health programs.* Washington, DC, Focus on Young Adults, 2000 (Focus Tool Series 3).

10. Glaser EM, Abelson HH, Garrison KN. *Putting knowledge to use.* San Francisco, CA, Jossey-Bass Inc., 1983.

11. Martin A, McEvoy M, Townsend JW. Approaches to strengthening the utilization of OR results: dissemination. In: Seidman M, Horn MC, eds. *Operations research: helping family planning programs work better.* New York, Wiley-Liss Inc., 1991:433–450.

12. Nutbeam N. Achieving "best practice" in health promotion: improving the fit between research and practice. *Health Education Research*, 1996, 11:317–326.

13. Bero LA, Grilli R, Grimshaw JM et al. Closing the gap between research and practice: an overview of systematic reviews of interventions to promote the implementation of research findings. *BMJ*, 1998, 317:465–468.

14. Haines A, Donald A. *Getting research findings into practice.* London, BMJ Books, 1998.

15. Porter RW. *Knowledge utilization and the process of policy formation – toward a framework for Africa.* Washington, DC, Academy for Educational Development, Support for Analysis and Research in Africa (SARA Project), 1999.

16. NHS Centre for Reviews and Dissemination. Getting evidence into practice. *Effective Health Care*, 1999, 5:1–16.

17. Stone D. Using knowledge: the dilemmas of bridging research and policy. *Compare*, 2002, 32:285–296.

18. Ogden J, Walt G, Lush L. The politics of "branding" in policy transfer: the case of DOTS for tuberculosis control. *Social Science and Medicine*, 2003, 57:179–188.

19. IIRR. *Going to scale: can we bring more benefits to more people more quickly?* Silan, Cavite, Philippines, International Institute of Rural Reconstruction, YC James Yen Center, 2000.

20. Guendel S, Jancock J, Anderson S. *Scaling-up strategies for research in natural resources management: a comparative review.* Chatham, University of Greenwich, Natural Resources Institute, 2001.

21. Simmons R, Hall P, Díaz J et al. The strategic approach to contraceptive introduction. *Studies in Family Planning*, 1997, 28:79–94.

22. Satia J, Fajans P, Elias C et al. A strategic approach to reproductive health programme development. *Asia-Pacific Population Journal*, 2000, 15:5–38.

23. *Strategic Approach.* Geneva, World Health Organization (http://www.who.int/reproductive-health/strategic_approach, accessed 27 March 2005).

24. Fajans P, Simmons R, Ghiron L. Helping public sector health systems innovate: the strategic approach to strengthening reproductive health policies and programs. *American Journal of Public Health*, 2006, 96:435–440.

Chapter 1

Scaling up health service innovations: a framework for action

Ruth Simmons[a], Jeremy Shiffman[b]

Summary

This chapter provides a conceptual framework for scaling up, with a focus on evidence-based reproductive health service innovations. It cites an extensive literature from several disciplines. The framework links an innovation to be scaled up with four other elements: a resource team that promotes it; a user organization expected to adopt the innovation; a strategy to transfer it; and an environment in which the transfer takes place. The authors discuss key attributes that have been found to facilitate the scaling-up process and identify strategic choices that must be made to ensure success. A final section identifies the diverse environments in which scaling up occurs, arguing that successful scale up requires tailoring strategies to the various dimensions of these settings.

Introduction

At times, good ideas spread of their own accord. They may be so ground-breaking, involve such pioneering technology and meet such pressing needs that they proliferate seamlessly from person to person, organization to organization and country to country. Most good ideas, however, do not spread with such ease. They require the backing and energies of committed individuals and organizations to design and carry out strategies for expansion that are carefully tailored to the realities of their settings. The question of sustainable scaling up is at issue,

[a] Ruth Simmons is Professor in the Department of Health Behavior and Health Education School of Public Health, University of Michigan.

[b] Jeremy Shiffman is Associate Professor of Public Administration in the Maxwell School of Syracuse University.

defined in this book as the effort to magnify the impact of health service innovations successfully tested in pilot or experimental projects, so as to benefit more people and to foster policy and programme development on a lasting basis[1]. The emphasis is on interventions that have been tested in the country context within which they will be scaled up.

With increasing interest in scaling up, efforts to identify and characterize its stages, processes and outcomes have begun to multiply (1, 3–9). There is no agreement on basic terms, concepts and typologies, but there are nonetheless extensive commonalities in the basic themes and conclusions that are being reached. We present here a conceptual framework for scaling up that builds on the insights from literature in a variety of relevant fields, the case-studies in this book, discussions from a series of meetings at the Rockefeller Foundation's Study and Conference Center in Bellagio, Italy, and the authors' experience. Our focus is on the wider use of health service innovations within public sector programmes, but the framework can also be applied to other contexts.

What we present is not a theory, in that it articulates no universal, testable set of propositions stating why scaling up may succeed or fail. Rather, it is a way of thinking about the process that identifies its primary components, the choices to be made and the circumstances that may facilitate or hamper effectiveness and sustainability. The framework links five elements: the innovation that has proven to be successful on a small scale; the individuals or institutions facilitating its wider use; the potential or actual users of the innovation; the strategies employed for having broader impact; and the context or environment in which all this takes place. Grounded in an open systems perspective, the framework emphasizes that scaling up is not an insulated process unaffected by the outside world. Instead, it is strongly shaped by external forces such as the pervasiveness of poverty in a country, the capacity of the broader national health system and its bureaucratic institutions, the specific health needs of populations, the degree of democratic political participation and global influences.

---

[1]   This definition is more specific than when scaling up is more broadly defined to refer to "increasing the socioeconomic impact from a small to a large scale of coverage" (1, p. 5), or the very broad and general definition of scaling up as "doing more" in a technical area of health or development (see for example 2). When scaling up refers to "the process of expanding the scale of activities with the ultimate objective of increasing the number of people and increasing the impact of the intervention with a specific objective of regularizing it into routine public sector health services (3, p. 22, citing Julie Solo of the Reproductive Health Alliance), it is very similar to the definition used here, except that we emphasize the availability of evidence that interventions have been successfully tested or evaluated in the local context in which they are to be implemented.

We reviewed literature from diverse fields – some of it published, some of it web-based, and some of it in unpublished "grey" form – to distil the considerable wisdom that exists. International health and family planning case-studies, while not numerous and some of them older, provide insights on scaling up in these sectors (key examples include *3, 9–20*). Discussion has been quite extensive in the rural development and natural resource management literatures, both of which aid in the identification of approaches to scaling up and the forms it takes (see for example *1, 4, 6, 21–24*). A key theme in these literatures has been the question of how nongovernmental organizations (NGOs) can expand their influence and enter into effective partnerships with government without losing their traditional flexibility and social change values[2]. Several decades of research on the diffusion of innovation, knowledge transfer and the integration of research into policy – although not explicitly focused on the concept of scaling up – point to factors that facilitate the widespread use of new practices.[3] Similarly, literature from the policy, organization and management sciences helped us to characterize the diverse contexts in which scaling up takes place, to articulate the strategic choices that must be made and to consider issues of planning, implementation and monitoring that are required for expanding innovations (*37–41*).

The discussion of the framework is divided into three parts: Part 1 presents the elements of the framework as well as attributes of success; Part 2 identifies key choices involved in planning a scaling-up strategy; and Part 3 reviews the range of environmental factors that must be taken into account. As we develop these ideas, we draw from and highlight the contributions of existing scholarship. The focus here is on the process of scaling up and on successful principles of practice. This chapter does not cover the measurement of outcomes and impacts, address the costs of scaling up[4], or provide step-by-step guidance on how to proceed.

---

[2] These concerns are well represented in *3, 14, 25*.

[3] Study of the diffusion of innovation and knowledge transfer began in the early 1940s. The diffusion of innovation and planned change were the subject of many publications. Although still pursued in the social sciences, these issues have become less prominent than they were in the 1960s, 1970s and early 1980s. However, related work has been done recently under such rubrics as research utilization and dissemination, putting knowledge into practice, bridging research and policy, etc. (See for example *19, 26–36*).

[4] For cost considerations in scaling up see Chapter 4 and *42*.

Part 1. The elements of scaling up and attributes of success

The process of going to scale occurs within a system of the following elements: the innovation, the resource organization or resource team, the user organization, the scaling-up strategy and the environment (Figure 1.1).

The **innovation** designates what is being scaled up. In this chapter and throughout the book it refers to health service interventions tested in pilot or experimental projects to improve equitable access to an appropriate range of care with good quality. In other settings the innovation may refer to new practices that are not focused on services. Following the lead of Rogers (29), we use the concept of innovation because these practices are new in the local contexts where they are being introduced. Rogers points out that it matters little whether the idea, practice or object is new or whether it is only perceived to be so. If it is perceived to be new, it is considered an innovation.[5] We use the term innovation as shorthand for a package of interventions, rather than a single intervention, including not only new service components but also the managerial processes necessary for successful implementation.

This book's focus is on family planning, related aspects of reproductive health and primary health care, working within the mandate of the agenda developed at the International Conference on Population and Development held in Cairo in 1994 (43) and the Millennium Declaration (44). Innovations involve organizing culturally appropriate outreach services or clinic-based interventions seeking to improve availability and access to care, technical competence, and interpersonal relations as well as to introduce the principle and practice of free and informed choice. Some of the interventions have incorporated strong gender, reproductive rights and empowerment perspectives. All the interventions emphasize listening to the voices of those affected by the services and involving them.[6]

The **resource organization or team** refers to the individuals and organizations that have been involved in the development and testing of the reproductive health innovations and/or seek to facilitate their wider use. Reproductive health advocates, researchers, programme

---

[5]   Cooley and Kohl prefer the term "model" (8).

[6]   Porter and Prysor-Jones have highlighted the importance of communication, stating that "research most effectively informs policy-making and management when there is a three-way process linking researchers, decision-makers and those most affected by whatever issues are under consideration" (31).

managers, trainers, service providers, community representatives and policy-makers are examples of people who may play such a catalytic role. They may be located in a variety of settings – nongovernmental or governmental organizations, research centres and technical assistance agencies. The resource organization/team also may consist of a network or coalition of individuals located in various institutions. A resource team may be situated in the same formal organization which seeks to, or is expected to adopt the innovation or it may be located outside of it. It may be formally charged with promoting the wider utilization of innovations or may act informally in this role.

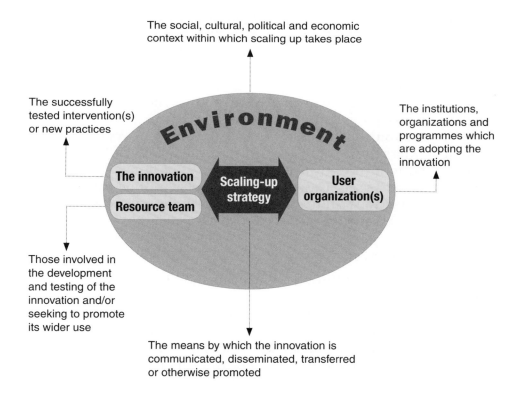

Figure 1.1 The elements of scaling up

The **user organization** refers to the institutions or organizations within which the innovations are expected to be widely adopted and implemented. In the case-studies in the following chapters, the user organizations are the health service systems at national, regional and local levels. The distinction between resource team and user organization is essential. It highlights the frequently invisible – though essential – role of the catalysts who promote and support the transfer of innovations and distinguishes it from those who are seeking to adopt them. Individuals may be members of both the resource organization/ team and the user organization. Moreover, strategic actors located in the user organization can become members of the resource team as they develop expertise and interest in supporting expansion.

The **scaling-up strategy** designates the means by which the innovation is communicated, transferred or otherwise promoted. This includes decisions about what exactly will be taken to scale; how the innovation will be disseminated; what type of scaling up will be appropriate; how it will be organized; how fast it will be pursued; how various environmental challenges and opportunities will be engaged; and what role research will play in the process. These various choices will be discussed in Part 2 and Part 3 of this chapter.

The **environment** of scaling up includes both the people and communities who require health services as well as the multiple actors, sectors and influences that shape the process of bringing successful interventions to scale. These include the policy setting, the political system, bureaucratic culture, the health sector, the socioeconomic and cultural contexts and the influence of global trends.

Attributes of success

Studies of the diffusion of innovation and knowledge transfer highlight key attributes that facilitate successful expansion of innovations. These attributes provide a parsimonious list of relevant factors that have been supported by much of the existing scaling-up literature. Attributes are here organized around the central elements of the framework depicted in Figure 1.1, namely the innovation, the resource team or organization, the user organization and the scaling-up strategy. Considerations relevant for the environment in which scaling up occurs will be discussed in Part 3.

Attributes of the innovation

Summarizing findings from multiple studies, Glaser and colleagues (26) identified seven characteristics that facilitate innovation transfer, many of which have also been reinforced by recent writing on research utilization. Innovations must be:

- based on sound evidence or espoused by respected persons or institutions in order to be **credible**;
- **observable** to ensure that potential users can see the results;
- **relevant** for addressing persistent or sharply felt problems;
- have a **relative advantage** over existing practices;
- **easy to install** and understand;
- **compatible** with the potential users' established values, norms and facilities;
- **testable** without committing the potential user to complete adoption.

The case-studies from China and Ghana in this book provide examples of how sound evidence plays a critical role in advancing the cause of scaling up. In China, advocates from both inside and outside the country carefully deployed information from an assessment of six quality-of-care pilot projects to promote broader reform in the national family planning programme (Chapter 3). In Ghana, information on health and fertility outcomes of a newly tested, community-based approach to service delivery was used at regional and national forums to demonstrate its effectiveness to policy-makers (Chapter 5). Other studies from the fields of international health and family planning have also demonstrated the critical role of sound evidence for effective scaling up (*11, 16*).

The nature of the evidence needed depends on the project's objectives as well as on the level of evidence demanded by those making decisions about scaling up. For instance, health service innovations that seek to affect fertility typically require population-based data on fertility or contraceptive prevalence. However, decision-makers may be satisfied with service statistics related to the provision of contraceptives. Innovations whose major purpose is to bring about changes in the quality of and access to reproductive health services do not necessarily require population-based data. They can demonstrate their effectiveness with information related to service functioning.

Pilot or experimental projects often introduce a range of innovations, not all of which are central to the initiative's success. An additional component of presenting credible evidence, therefore, is to document which aspects of the interventions were most central in producing the desired results, which can then also make it possible to simplify the innovation. For a more extensive discussion of this point see Cooley and Kohl (*8*) and Chapter 4.

When pilot or experimental projects are tested in social and managerial environments that differ greatly from the setting into which they are to be transferred, a second research phase may be called for in which the innovations are validated in more typical programmatic contexts before large-scale expansion proceeds (see Chapters 5 and 6).

Transfer of projects from one setting to another is facilitated when innovations are easy to install, there is obvious demand for them, they are not costly and/or the resources for their introduction are available, and their implementation does not require much time. As the case-studies reported in this book indicate, however, the service interventions that are required to improve access, quality and the range of reproductive health services do not necessarily meet these criteria. The innovations discussed here differ considerably from existing service delivery practices. They all imply a significant degree of change, requiring technical assistance and other resources to ensure implementation. Moreover, as the Viet Nam experience shows, when some components of an intervention are easier to install than others tensions may result over which of them should be the focus of scaling up (Chapter 2).

If innovations are not compatible with the user organization's practices and aims, scaling up will be difficult. For example, in a nutrition project in India, conflict between the NGO and the government contributed to the project's failure (*10*). In another instance, when advocates in a family planning intervention in Bangladesh threatened existing power relationships by taking steps to eliminate bureaucratic irregularities, the programme stalled (*15*).

Attributes of the resource team

The literature on the diffusion of innovation and knowledge transfer does not focus on the characteristics of the resource team that lead to successful transfer; the attributes presented here are based on general insights from the social and political entrepreneurship and organization behaviour literature as well as on lessons from the case-studies in this book. Resource teams involved in the promotion of the innovation are more likely to be successful if they possess the following features:

- effective and motivated **leaders** who command authority and have credibility with the user organization;
- a unifying **vision**;
- an **appreciation of the user organization's** capacities and limitations;
- an **understanding** of the political, social and cultural environments within which scaling up takes place;
- the ability to generate financial and technical **resources**;

- relevant **technical skills**;
- **training capacity**;
- **management skills**.

Resource teams must act with entrepreneurship and ability to promote innovations in constrained environments. These teams are more likely to be successful when they have effective leaders who are able to inspire team members to embrace and pursue well-defined goals.[7] Ideally, such individuals are persistent, well connected, have coalition-building skills, articulate a clear vision amidst complexity and have credibility that facilitates the mobilization of resources. It is also desirable for them to know how to generate commitment by appealing to social values; to identify the critical challenges in their environments; and to have management skills, training capacity and relevant technical competence. The importance of such effective leadership as a critical element in scaling up was identified in an analysis of BRAC's programmes in Bangladesh (*51*).

Attributes of the user organization

The user organization refers here to public-sector institutions responsible for the provision of health services. According to the diffusion of innovation literature (*26*), successful transfer of innovations is facilitated when the user organization has the following characteristics:

- the members of the user organization **perceive a need for the innovation**;
- the user organization has the appropriate **implementation capacity**;
- the **timing** and circumstances are right;
- the user organization possesses effective **leadership** and internal advocacy;
- the resource and user organizations are **similar in characteristics** and are in close physical proximity.

Public-sector health systems rarely have the ideal characteristics for scaling up health service innovations focused on equitable access, quality of care and an appropriate range of services (*52*). Working in hierarchical systems that emphasize rules, control and order, mid-level public servants may not perceive the need for improvements in quality of care or may not have the necessary implementation capacity.

---

[7] A long line of scholarship on political and social entrepreneurship identifies the features of entrepreneurial leaders that are able to enact change, for example see *45–50*.

New practices involve careful listening, patience, time and a respectful, non-hierarchical mode of communication between providers and clients. Meanwhile, managers and providers want clear, measurable, immediate results. They are besieged by multiple priorities and face a perpetual shortage of resources to respond to them. Implementing the Cairo agenda requires major change in bureaucratic culture.

Resource teams must therefore temper expectations in accordance with the realities of the user organization. In settings where political leaders are committed to reproductive health, where national health systems are strong and health personnel competent, rapid large scale expansion of innovations may be feasible. In others, where national leaders look unfavourably upon reproductive health or accord it low priority, health systems are weak, or the political system is decentralized and power fragmented, scaling-up proponents may need to set realistic expectations about how much can be accomplished.

Past research demonstrates that relationships between resource teams and user organizations are dynamic rather than static (53). Each influences the other, and the resource team itself is changed as it engages in the process of bringing innovations to scale. Moreover, members of the user organization may become part of the resource team as they acquire familiarity and expertise with the innovation. The Reprolatina Project in Latin America, an initiative to build training capacity at the municipal level within the public sector, illustrates this dynamism (Chapter 8), as does a nutrition programme in Viet Nam where local villagers who gained expertise in the programme during its initial testing then became a resource for other villages in the process of expansion (54).

Attributes of the scaling-up strategy

Diffusion of innovation research and other literature on scaling up indicate that successful transfer is more likely to occur when the scaling-up strategy has the following characteristics:

- **clear messages** through which the advantages of the innovation are made visible;
- **personal contact** and informal communication;
- **early involvement** of members of the user organization;
- **adaptation** of the innovation to the local context;
- **participatory** approaches;
- **technical assistance** and a supportive approach;
- **sufficient time** to implement new approaches;
- **strong diffusion channels**;
- **training support** to ensure skills transfer;

- systematic use of **evidence** on the process and outcomes of scaling up;
- ongoing focus on **sustainability**.

Academic jargon and the lengthy and technical nature of research reports constitute barriers to the dissemination of findings. Mediation between researchers and the user organization is sometimes necessary to bridge this gap. Personal contact with decision-makers is also critical (55). For example, briefings for policy-makers that employ clear messages tailored to their specific needs can facilitate innovation transfer. Resource teams need to identify key players of the user organization, understand their needs, engage them in the design of pilot projects, and involve them in analysis of project results (56). At the same time they must continue to engage with the communities and people for whose benefit innovations have been designed, thus linking the resource team, the user organization and beneficiaries in a three-way process of communication (31). Studies on international health and family planning emphasize the importance of technical assistance and of a long time frame to facilitate transfer (see for example 11, 15, 16). Governments often lack training and management support to implement quality of care (57). Research on reproductive health programmes repeatedly finds that preparation of training teams and materials and provision of continuous training is needed for successful scaling up (see for example 15–17, 54 and Chapter 8).

Part 2. Strategic choices in planning a scaling-up strategy

Scaling up involves strategic choices along many dimensions. Here we discuss key decisions related to: the type of scaling up used; the process of communicating the innovation and preparing users in its application; the organizational options selected in implementing the process; assessing costs and resource mobilization; and monitoring and researching the process and outcomes of scaling up (see Figure 1.2).

Decisions about these strategic choices must be made in light of the opportunities and challenges presented by the various environments within which scaling up takes place. They must take into account the policy and political context, the characteristics of the health sector, the bureaucratic culture within which it operates and the socioeconomic and cultural factors that shape people's needs and rights. The influence of these larger environmental factors and the need to strategize how best to navigate them is discussed in Part 3.

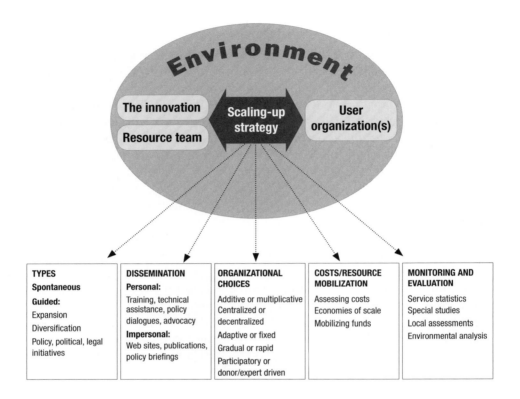

Figure 1.2 Strategic choices in scaling up

Types of scaling up

Sceptics might argue that sustained attention to scaling up is unnecessary. Ample evidence exists that innovations spread spontaneously from individual to individual and from innovative programme settings to other environments. Gladwell has argued that relatively small changes can produce a "tipping point" (58), where innovative behaviour becomes so contagious that it spreads like outbreaks of infectious disease. Such **spontaneous diffusion** has been observed in health as well as in other fields (52, 59). The advantage of spontaneous diffusion of innovation is obvious: much effort and cost are spared in organizing and guiding scaling-up initiatives. These advantages make it worthwhile to evaluate whether deliberate scaling-up efforts can be tailored to facilitate the spontaneous spread of health service innovations. The China case-study in Chapter 3 provides examples of the power of spontaneous diffusion of family planning service innovations. In cases of such spontaneous expansion, however, it is important to ensure that the essence of the innovation remains intact. Incomplete or superficial transfer can compromise the results.

Despite examples where spontaneous diffusion of innovation has occurred, in most cases deliberate attention to scaling up is essential. Without guidance or deliberate fostering most small-scale research-based improvements in health services have failed to lead to policy and programme development. Three different paths of deliberate or **guided scaling up** may be pursued: replication or expansion, also referred to as horizontal scaling up; diversification; and political, policy or legal initiatives, also referred to as vertical scaling up (6).[8] Expansion or horizontal scaling up occurs when innovations are replicated in different locations or are expanded to serve larger populations or different categories of beneficiaries (5, 22).[9] Diversification, also referred to as functional scaling up or grafting, consists of testing and adding new interventions to existing innovations (see for example 17, 22). Vertical or political scaling up takes place when innovations are institutionalized through policy or legal action. Systems and structures are adapted and resources redistributed to build the institutional mechanisms that can ensure sustainability.

The different types of scaling up do not function in isolation. Spontaneous diffusion may occur in combination with scaling up that is guided, and expansion is typically most effective when supported by political and institutional scaling up. This point has been widely emphasized in the literature (5, 6, 21, 25, 57, 60).

Dissemination approaches

Impersonal communications strategies, such as academic publications, policy briefs, web sites, manuals, guides, tool kits and other forms of documentation, are essential for dissemination but by them-

---

[8]   The literature does not present a consistent use of typologies for scaling up. Authors who have discussed these particular types are Clark (21), Edwards and Hulme (25); and Uvin and Miller (22).

[9]   Cooley and Kohl distinguish between replication and expansion, viewing the former as "increasing the scale of operations of the organization that originally developed and piloted the model" and the latter as "increasing the use of a particular process, technology or model of service delivery by getting other organizations … to take up and implement the model" (8). In the framework presented here such organizational issues are distinguished as additive or multiplicative organizational choices. Some authors prefer the term expansion because replication implies mechanical, franchise models to scaling up which are considered less valuable for the type of scaling up discussed here.

selves are insufficient to scale up health service innovations. Personal communication and support in the form of training programmes, site visits, workshops, conferences, policy forums or dialogues, supportive supervision and technical support are needed (31, 32, 53). Approaches may vary in length of time commitment from relatively short-term activities to more extensive ones supporting organization development efforts in the utilization and adaptation of the innovation.

The specific choice of dissemination approach will depend on the nature of the innovation and the capacity of the user organization to absorb the implied changes. As demonstrated by the case-studies from Viet Nam (Chapter 2) and Brazil (Chapter 8), when the amount of change implied by the innovation is large, the technical, supervisory and training support required can be extensive, often requiring well-resourced organization development approaches.

Organizational choices

Scaling-up practitioners are faced with many organizational choices as they seek to promote the wider utilization of health service innovations. Key options discussed in the literature are: (1) additive versus multiplicative strategies; (2) centralized, top-down versus decentralized bottom-up approaches; (3) flexible, adaptive strategies versus implementation of a standard package of interventions; (4) gradual versus rapid implementation; and (5) participatory versus expert or management-dominated approaches.

The distinction between **additive and multiplicative strategies** – also referred to as direct and indirect strategies (1) – has been made in the development literature (25, 61). A strategy is additive when the original sponsor or sponsors of the innovation are the ones who plan and implement the scaling-up effort. When new partners join in the expansion and promotion of the innovation, the strategy is multiplicative. The distinction between additive and multiplicative strategies draws attention to the need for building the institutional capacity to support scaling-up initiatives. The additive approach places the full organizational burden of implementing the scaling-up initiative on one organization or supporting it by relying on a single resource team. Multiplicative strategies distribute the burden across several organizations. The term "association" has been used to describe a multiplicative strategy of piecing together coverage obtained from several projects (14).

While involving multiple partners in scaling up has much potential, it does not come without cost. For example, the Reprolatina Project recognized early on that building capacity for training others in the process of expanding health service innovations was essential (see Chapter 8). However, developing training capacity is time-consuming and frustrating when trainers are transferred or for other reasons leave their positions, or when changes in political leadership lead to withdrawal of support for newly trained staff (62). The choice of a multiplicative strategy also involves the need for a shared philosophy and vision among partners, in the absence of which much time can be lost in reaching consensus or compromise rather than advancing towards goals.

If scaling-up initiatives are directed by a **central authority** – for example, a ministry of health – it is possible to mandate large-scale replication. The role of such a central mandate is discussed in Chapter 5, comparing the experience of Bangladesh and Ghana. Centralized scaling-up initiatives, though powerful, may also be constrained by the penchant of central authorities to mandate rigid implementation of a new service model, making it difficult to ensure that innovations are appropriately adapted to local contexts. In contrast, **decentralized approaches** allow local initiative, autonomy, spontaneity, mutual learning and problem-solving (23, 57). Their obvious disadvantage is that they do not have the reach of central authorities, and often do not command sufficient influence or resources to ensure appropriate policy reform. Furthermore, local autonomy may lead to the loss of essential features of the tested innovations.

The literature of various disciplines stresses the importance of **adaptive strategies and flexibility**, arguing, for example, that organizations with a capacity to learn are more likely to succeed in whatever they choose to do than organizations that are rigidly bound by rules and emphasize standardization. The important role of learning organizations (24, 40, 63) has also been highlighted in discussions of scaling up (1) because the environments of scaling up differ extensively from country to country, province to province and even from one district to another. In one country the social environment may suggest a social mobilization and a community-based strategy. In another, stronger reliance on the formal institutions of the state may be more relevant (13). Thus, adaptation and learning continue to be essential as scaling up proceeds (17, 20, 54).

As they are adapted locally, innovations may be simplified, thereby shortening the time required for implementation and moving from a concern about effectiveness to one of efficiency (16, 24). At the same time, essential ingredients responsible for the success of the innovative package must be maintained sufficiently intact to ensure success.

While context-specific adaptation is essential, universal principles have their place as well. For example, the eligibility criteria for contraceptive use that have been established according to internationally agreed standards must not be changed locally. Also, such normative principles as free and informed choice and reproductive rights should be viewed as universal requirements rather than as open to opportunistic local interpretation. However, the China case-study in Chapter 3 shows that local adaptation of these concepts may constitute a significant advance. Thus, we agree with Wazir & van Oudenhoven who conclude that "a sensitive balance has to be struck between accepting what is universal or global while recognizing and protecting what is valuable at the local level" (23).

Another strategic choice concerns the pace of scaling up. Innovations may be expanded in a **phased or gradual manner** or they may be rapidly scaled up. Some authors refer to **rapid implementation** as explosive scaling up (14). The literature generally emphasizes the importance of gradual approaches, citing the importance of learning by doing, and having the requisite time to adapt the innovation to local circumstances (15). In reviewing the determinants of successful development initiatives in several countries, Paul identified "phased implementation" as a major ingredient of success (39). Orienting public sector bureaucracies, so that they maximize the individual well-being of each person who receives care and adhere to a philosophy of reproductive health more generally, is not a task that can be accomplished quickly. The need to institutionalize this philosophy may be in tension with another principle, discussed below in Part 3: the value of taking advantage of policy windows. A politically opportune moment may arise when advocates can place reproductive health on the agenda; taking advantage of such a moment, however, may mean loss of control by the resource team over the speed of implementation. Such a trade-off occurred in Viet Nam (Chapter 2).

A final organizational choice relates to the distinction between **participatory approaches** and **strategies dominated by experts, donors or management**. Participation is such an essential component of the Cairo reproductive health paradigm that it carries both normative and practical weight. Apart from being a valued end in itself, participation of all relevant stakeholders (including women's health advocates and other community members) can increase the probability that local needs are appropriately reflected upon and taken into account (62). Participation mobilizes a broader range of support for the resource team and the user organization than would otherwise be available. The importance of using participatory approaches has been strongly emphasized in the scaling-up literature (for example 16, 17, 24, 31, 54, 57, 64). However, the human and financial costs of large-scale participation are considerable and may therefore constrain the degree of involvement that is feasible. For example, ministries of health are limited in their capacity to mobilize communities. Therefore extensive participation may be difficult to sustain (*14*).

Assessing costs and mobilizing resources

The fourth area of strategic decision-making relates to costs and resource mobilization. Costs arise for all types of scaling up: 1) for expanding the innovation to new geographical sites or population groups; 2) for the often considerable time and effort needed to obtain political support and for advocacy to institutionalize the innovation; 3) for diversifying the innovation through the additional testing and implementation of new components; and 4) for evaluating and working with spontaneous scaling up that may arise. Knowing the costs involved is key to the formulation of a scaling-up strategy.

Scaling up does not necessarily require the infusion of massive external funding; in fact it is critical to explore what options exist to minimize the additional resources that will be needed. Can the user organization take on the innovation using resources available from within the health system? Are economies of scale possible - for example by connecting the innovation to related efforts or through creative ways of resource sharing? However, because scaling up is not a routine process, some dedicated resources or donor support are necessary until implementation of the innovation becomes a standard practice and its costs are fully included in national and local budgets. Linking the innovation to macro-level funding mechanisms such as Sector-wide Approaches may be an important approach towards mobilizing such support (*65*).

Monitoring and evaluation

Successful scaling up requires the systematic use of evidence to guide the process and incorporate new learning. Existing systems of monitoring and evaluating service delivery are rarely capable of capturing issues relevant to the process and outcomes of moving to scale. Special research and evaluation procedures should monitor whether the innovation is being implemented as expected and the extent to which local adaptation maintains minimum established standards. Plans and resources for further expansion can be adjusted when problems and dysfunctions are encountered. At the same time, identifying the positive features and results obtained from scaling up motivates communities, providers, decision-makers and managers by demonstrating the value of new approaches. The need for greater scientific understanding of the determinants of successful scaling up provides an additional important reason for special attention to researching the process.

Part 3. Navigating diverse environments when scaling up

Strategic choices for broadening the impact of health service innovations have to be made within a larger socioeconomic, political, cultural and institutional context. Although the ideal conditions do not exist anywhere, most socioeconomic, cultural and bureaucratic environments are likely to offer some opportunities for scaling up. The major challenge is to identify where such opportunities exist and to make strategic choices about how to proceed, seeking to optimize strengths and minimize constraints. The strategic management literature suggests analysis of these external conditions should be undertaken early on in the planning process.[10] Planning should focus on creating congruence among key elements of the scaling-up process. We turn to this task next, describing the range of environments relevant for ensuring broader impact of health service innovations (see Figure 1.3).

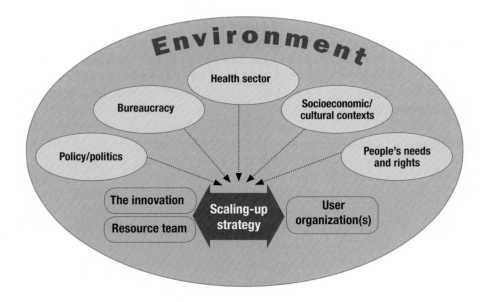

Figure 1.3 The diverse environments of scaling up

---

[10] For examples see *37–39, 41*; for an example from the scaling-up literature see *3*.

Policy setting and political context

Many issues compete for priority at international and national levels, while only a few receive attention. Political scientists have termed such sorting of issues the "agenda-setting" phase of the public policy process (46). The 1994 International Conference on Population and Development, held in Cairo, represents an example of successful agenda setting. An alliance of governments, international organizations and NGOs brought global attention to reproductive health, creating an international policy window for the cause. This attention in turn shaped national policy priorities. Chapter 3 explains how members of the Chinese State Family Planning Commission attended the Cairo Conference, learned of the new paradigm and convinced their Minister to permit pilot projects in quality of care.

Such policy windows open only for limited periods of time. In an environment of scarce resources for health and of transient policy windows, advocates for scaling up reproductive health service innovations must think strategically to ensure the sustainability of the cause. When policy windows are open, the questions of how to sustain the stimulus once the window closes should be considered early on. Newly elected or appointed decision-makers typically wish to impose their own imprint upon the policy scene and, for a variety of reasons, rarely maintain programmes initiated by their predecessors.

The nature of the national political system will also shape scaling-up choices. In democracies many actors influence reproductive health priorities, including parliamentarians who may introduce legislation on reproductive health and nongovernmental organizations involved in programmes and advocacy. In less democratic settings, governments often curtail the power of these actors, concentrating authority in the hands of public servants and military officials. The network of actors that scaling-up proponents must target in order to promote their causes will therefore vary by the type of political structure.

Bureaucratic culture

Public sector bureaucracies implement the policies enacted by national political bodies. Understanding the institutions within which policies are implemented is therefore also critical for shaping appropriate scaling-up strategies. Many are slow, infused with political interests, beholden by layers of rules, averse to taking risks, prone to seek immediate and simple solutions to complex problems, staffed with poorly paid civil servants who cannot survive on their public salaries alone, and subject to frequent personnel changes (66). Bureaucracies vary in the degree to which they exercise authority and engage with various social sectors (*67*): some have considerable authority and are able to get things done; others have minimal legitimacy and accomplish little. At times, they act as efficient, rational implementers of national policy; more often, though, policy is altered in the process of implementation and sometimes it is not implemented at all. Effectiveness varies even within the same bureaucratic system: pockets of innovation exist alongside spheres of inefficiency, and policy entrepreneurs able to mobilize national political systems work beside unmotivated and ineffective public servants.

Given this variation, it is essential to understand the characteristics of the bureaucratic organizations responsible for scaling up reproductive health innovations. In particular, it is important to diagnose constraints as well as enabling factors from the outset and to avoid simplistic assumptions that bureaucracies have no interests of their own. Also, there is value in identifying innovative departments and policy entrepreneurs (*45–47, 50, 68*), for it is they who move systems.

Characteristics of the health sector

The health sector environment also shapes scaling-up possibilities. Health ministries tend to be among the weakest ministries in developing countries. The health portfolio is often handed to junior coalition partners in parliamentary systems or to politically weaker members of the regime, and health sectors typically command only a small percentage of national budgets. This is not to say that health causes cannot generate significant national attention. It does mean, however, that political coalitions frequently need to be constructed to incorporate actors outside the government health sector – often including finance ministry officials, prominent domestic social actors, donors and international NGOs – in order to generate political priority for scaling up health service innovations.

A second feature in many health systems is instability in leadership. Elections and political manoeuvering bring with them changes in national, regional and local health officials. As health leadership shifts, so may health priorities and the attention given to the effort to expand small-scale health service innovations. The case of Brazil in Chapter 7 illustrates the difficulties advocates can have in bringing service innovations to scale because of frequent changes in municipal-level leaders.

Apart from these long-standing institutional features of health sectors, a new issue has emerged: health sector reform. National leaders are streamlining and privatizing components of health systems seeking improved efficiency and better health outcomes, particularly for the poor (*7, 69*). These reforms have led to new uncertainties for the health sector, and often involve leadership changes and shifting policy priorities (*70*). As discussed in Chapter 4, for example, a health sector reform programme in Zambia created job instability among civil servants and interfered with activities designed to expand contraceptive choices.

A related change is decentralization. In the past decade, national governments have transferred varying degrees of decision-making and financial authority to local officials in order to make localities more responsive to the demands and needs of citizens (*71, 72*). This reform complicates scaling-up prospects because it increases considerably the number of decision-makers involved in setting health priorities. In more centralized systems, only a handful of leaders must agree in order to generate consensus for the national scaling up of health service innovations. In decentralized systems, scaling-up advocates may need to secure the agreement of hundreds of local-level decision-makers. Often authority is legally decentralized but central governments retain hold of funds, thereby making it difficult for local leaders to pursue their priorities.

There exist different kinds of decentralization (*40*), and analysts of health sector reform have distinguished among several types (*71, 73*). Scaling-up advocates must pay attention to the kind of decentralization that takes place, in order to determine who has gained and who has lost power to make policy and programmatic decisions.

The chapters in this book describe several instances of how decentralization shaped scaling-up strategies. For example, the Brazilian case-study in Chapter 7 shows that, because decision-making authority had been transferred to municipalities, the resource team had to target its strategies at politically appointed local health officials rather than working at the national or state level.

Socioeconomic and cultural contexts

Socioeconomic and cultural factors influence scaling-up prospects in multiple ways. They shape the need as well as the demand for health service innovations, and they also suggest appropriate ways to organize service delivery. How social forces shape both the demand for and supply of services is a question that must be taken into account at the stage of developing and testing health innovations. Social and cultural forces also create opportunities and constraints for bringing service innovations to scale. These possibilities must be carefully evaluated, assessing how the influence of social and cultural factors can be harnessed to magnify the impact of health service innovations tested in pilot or experimental projects.

Family planning programme research suggests that among the socioeconomic and cultural factors that may shape possibilities for scaling up reproductive health service innovations are: the strength of social networks; the receptivity of local and national religious leaders to reproductive health causes; the power of women of reproductive age in relation to other members of the household; local leadership structures; linguistic and ethnic differences between clients and service providers; and individual household resources and capacities to afford services. Chapter 6 notes that strong social networks in Ghana facilitated expansion of the Navrongo experiment, while weak social networks in Bangladesh necessitated reliance on the bureaucracy for scaling up. Chapter 7 shows how the opposition of the Catholic Church created difficulties for the scaling up of reproductive health innovations in Brazil.

Reproductive health needs, people's rights and perspectives

Seeking input and feedback from community members, including women, young people, men and others potentially affected by the innovation, gives voice to people's needs and concerns. Understanding their perceptions of costs, availability, potential side-effects and the manner in which clients are treated in health facilities is required in order to develop and expand innovations effectively. When women go to a health facility, they may be treated with scorn and disrespect. Thus the innovation often needs to include interventions that contribute to empowering people to insist on their rights.

Finally, the reproductive health status of the population constitutes an essential factor that must be evaluated not only at the stage of developing the innovation but as scaling up proceeds. One reason is that reproductive health needs vary by locality. For instance, a pilot project addressing sexually transmitted diseases may focus on adults. However, if adolescents also require such services in areas where scaling up occurs, strategies must be adapted to cover their needs as well. Assessing reproductive health attitudes and behaviour in target areas, including user perspectives on health technologies and health services, is therefore an essential step in the analysis of the scaling-up environment.

In sum, bringing health service innovations to scale occurs in an environment of intersecting global, national, bureaucratic, health sector, socioeconomic, political/policy and cultural forces. These do not form a simple, stable structure. They comprise a moving target, one that must be considered carefully if scaling up is to succeed. These environments necessarily condition how high to set one's goals and how fast they can be accomplished.

Conclusions

Scaling up health service innovations in public sector settings is a complex undertaking. We have sought to facilitate the process by providing a conceptual framework that links an innovation to be scaled up with four other elements: a resource team that facilitates its expansion; a user organization expected to adopt it; a strategy to transfer it; and an environment in which the transfer takes place.

These environments are diverse. Scaling up occurs in poor and prosperous countries; under democratic and autocratic regimes; in religious and secular societies; within bureaucracies that are honest and those infused with corruption; in settings where donor funding is available and in others where it is extremely limited. Advocates must therefore tailor their strategy to the realities of their settings and avoid the expectation that going to scale will proceed smoothly from research to action (15). The real world is disorderly. Scaling up health service innovations will require that advocates appreciate this disorder and that they decipher how to navigate it. The attributes of success and the strategic choices outlined in this chapter can be helpful tools in this process.

Those who seek to bring health service innovations to scale confront several key risks. The resources to move forward may not be available or changes in the managerial, political or policy environment may disfavour continued attention to scaling up. In addition, the process may be much more complex than anticipated. Moreover, as broader coverage is obtained, service innovations may begin to lose their essential humanistic and quality-of-care components (3, 14, 15, 24), may sacrifice their participatory characteristics, or may not be sustainable at all. There are no easy ways of addressing these risks; however four principles for successful practice emerge from the extensive experience that has been accumulated.

First, it is essential to begin with the end in mind. Concerns for scaling up should be a key consideration when pilot or experimental projects are designed, rather than being a second generation of issues to be considered when research is completed. Although early attention cannot solve all future problems, it begins to lay the groundwork for sustainable scaling up by involving future decision-makers and taking into account the resource environment in which expansion is to take place.

Second, a strong resource team which has forged close ties to local communities is the best guarantee that scaling-up initiatives will be assured sustainability and success. A dedicated and competent resource team with staying power can weather bad times, reconfigure strategic choices and move forward as new policy windows open and organizational obstacles diminish or disappear.

Third, and perhaps most importantly, it is essential to strive for a scaling-up strategy that achieves balance or congruence among the innovation, the resource team, the user organization and the environment. When the elements are out of balance, the number of obstacles to be confronted will be greatly increased. At the same time, scaling-up advocates must recognize that in reality such balance is neither easy to achieve nor always feasible. As illustrated by several of the case-studies in this book, attempts to balance the relative strengths and weaknesses among the elements may result in compromise but can also suggest creative ways of designing scaling-up strategies.

Finally, attention to research and evaluation with a focus on both the process and impact of moving to scale is essential. This contrasts with the common presumption that scaling up is a routine task and does not require special monitoring or assessment. Continued attention to evaluation and even to the appropriate methodologies for such evaluation is critical to assess impact and develop clearer understanding of the determinants of successful scaling up. Standard monitoring devices often do not provide information on the more qualitative and humanistic dimensions of many of the innovations in reproductive health services. New and better indicators may need to be used, if not in routine service statistics then at least in special studies. Moreover, when experimental or pilot projects are organized under conditions that vary extensively from the scaling-up environment, additional small-scale validation may be needed to generate will and credibility.

The case studies in this book illustrate the concepts and issues presented in this framework and show how in each setting different approaches and strategies produce success and how each context generates its own set of barriers. However, the underlying principles of scaling-up practice and the commitment to building equitable access and quality of care in health services are remarkably similar.

Acknowledgements

We are grateful for the opportunity to discuss the ideas presented in this paper with participants in three meetings at the Rockefeller Foundation's Bellagio Study and Conference Center, and wish to thank the World Health Organization, the Bill and Melinda Gates Foundation and the University of Michigan for their financial support.

References

1. *Scaling up the impact of good practices in rural development: a working paper to support implementation of the World Bank's rural development strategy.* Washington, DC, The World Bank, 2003 (Agriculture and Rural Development Department, Report No. 26031).

2. Curran J, Debas H, Arya M et al., eds. *Scaling up treatment for the global AIDS pandemic: challenges and opportunities.* Washington, DC, Institute of Medicine of the National Academies, National Academies Press, 2004.

3. DeJong J. *Making an impact in HIV and AIDS – NGO experiences of scaling up.* London, ITDG Publishing, 2003.

4. Guendel S, Jancock J, Anderson S. *Scaling up strategies for research in natural resources management: a comparative review.* Chatham, Natural Resources Institute, 2001.

5. Uvin P. Fighting hunger at the grassroots: paths to scaling up. *World Development*, 1995, 23:927–940.

6. *Going to scale: can we bring more benefits to more people more quickly?* Silan, Cavite, Philippines, International Institute of Rural Reconstruction, YC James Yen Center, 2000.

7. Binswanger HP, Aiyar SS. *Scaling up community-driven development: theoretical underpinnings and program design implications.* Washington, DC, the World Bank, 2003 (World Bank Policy Research Working Paper No. 3039).

8. Cooley L, Kohl R. *Scaling up – a conceptual and operational framework.* Washington, DC, Management Services International, 2005 (http://www.msiworldwide.com/documents/ScalingUp.pdf, accessed 15 March 2006).

9. *Scaling up series: ten dimensions of scaling up reproductive health programs.* Arlington, VA, Advance Africa, 2002 (http://www.advanceafrica.org/publications_and_presentations/Technical_Papers/index.html, accessed 17 March 2005).

10. Pyle DF. From pilot project to operational program in India: the problems of transition. In: Grindle MS, ed. *Politics and policy implementation in the Third World.* Princeton, NJ, Princeton University Press, 1980.

11. Cernada GP. *Knowledge into action: a guide to research utilization.* Farmingdale, NY, Baywood Publishing Company, Inc., 1982.

12. Phillips JF, Simmons R, Simmons GB et al. Transferring health and family planning services innovations to the public sector: an experiment in organization development in Bangladesh. *Studies in Family Planning*, 1984, 15:62–73.

13. Phillips JF, Nyonator F, Barkat-e-Khuda et al. *Utilizing field experiments for evidence-based health program development in Bangladesh and Ghana: implications for HIV/AIDS programs in resource-constrained settings.* Paper presented at: Global Conference on HIV/AIDS, Barcelona, Spain, July 2002.

14. Myers RG. *The twelve who survive: strengthening programmes of early childhood development in the third world.* London and New York, Routledge, 1992.

15. Haaga JG, Maru RM. The effect of operations research on program changes in Bangladesh. *Studies in Family Planning*, 1996, 27:76–87.

16. Gonzales F, Arteaga E, Howard-Grabman L. Scaling up the WARMI project: lessons learned. In: Burkhalter BR, Graham VL, eds. *Presented papers: high impact PVO child survival programs*, Vol. 2. Proceedings of an Expert Consultation, Gallaudet University, 21–24 June 1998. Arlington, VA, CORE Group/BASICS Project/USAID, 1999.

17. Smith J, Colvin C. *Getting to scale in young adults reproductive health programs.* Washington, DC, Focus on Young Adults, 2000 (Focus Tool Series 3).

18. Huntington D, Nawar L. Moving from research to program – the Egyptian postabortion care initiative. *International Family Planning Perspectives*, 2003, 29:121–125.

19. Marin CM, Gage A, Khan S. *Frontiers in reproductive health.* New Orleans, LA, Tulane University, 2004 (unpublished).

20. Awoonor-Williams JK, Feinglass ES, Tobey R et al. Bridging the gap between evidence-based innovation and national health-sector reform in Ghana. *Studies in Family Planning*, 2004, 35:161–177.

21. Clark J. *Democratizing development.* Bloomfield, CT, Kumarian Press, 1991.

22. Uvin P, Miller D. Paths to scaling up: alternative strategies for local nongovernmental organizations. *Human Organization*, 1996, 55:344–354.

23. Wazir R, van Oudenhoven N. Increasing the coverage of social programmes. *International Social Science Journal*, 1998, 155:145–154.

24. Korten DC, Klauss R, eds. *People-centered development: contributions toward theory and planning frameworks*. West Hartford, CT, Kumarian Press, 1984.

25. Edwards M, Hulme D, eds. *Making a difference: NGOs and development in a changing world*. London, Earthscan Publications Ltd, 1992.

26. Glaser EM, Abelson HH, Garrison KN. *Putting knowledge to use: facilitating the diffusion of knowledge and the implementation of planned change*. San Francisco, CA, Jossey-Bass Inc., 1983.

27. Martin A, McEvoy M, Townsend JW (1991). Approaches to strengthening the utilization of OR results: dissemination. In: Seidman M, Horn MC, eds. *Operations research: helping family planning programs work better*. New York, Wiley-Liss Inc, 1991:433–450.

28. Porter RW, Hicks U. *Knowledge utilization and the process of policy formation – toward a framework for Africa*. Washington, DC, Academy for Educational Development, Support for Analysis and Research in Africa (SARA Project), 1995.

29. Rogers EM. *Diffusion of innovations*, 4th ed. New York, Free Press, 1995.

30. Nutbeam N. Achieving "best practice" in health promotion: improving the fit between research and practice. *Health Education Research*, 1996, 11:317–326.

31. Porter RW, Prysor-Jones S. *Making a difference to policies and programs: a guide for researchers*. Washington, DC, Academy for Educational Development, Support for Analysis and Research in Africa (SARA Project), 1997.

32. Bero LA, Grilli R, Grimshaw JM et al. Closing the gap between research and practice: an overview of systematic reviews of interventions to promote the implementation of research findings. *BMJ*, 1998, 317:465–468.

33. Haines A, Donald A. *Getting research findings into practice*. London, BMJ Books, 1998.

34. Crewe E, Young J. *Bridging research and policy: context, evidence and links*. London, Overseas Development Institute, 2002.

35. Stone D. Using knowledge: the dilemmas of "bridging research and policy". *Compare*, 2002, 32:285–296.

36. *Network: research to practice*. Research Triangle Park, NC, Family Health International, 2003.

37. Lawrence PR, Lorsch JW. *Organization and environment*. Homewood, IL, Irwin Inc, 1969.

38. Katz D, Kahn RL. *The social psychology of organizations*. New York, John Wiley and Sons, 1978.

39. Paul S. *Managing development programs: the lessons of success*. Boulder, CO, Westview Press, 1982.

40. Rondinelli DA, Nellis JR, Cheema GS. *Decentralization in developing countries: a review of recent experiences*. Washington, DC, The World Bank, 1983.

41. Donaldson L. *The contingency theory of organizations*. Thousand Oaks, CA, Sage Publications (Foundations for Organizational Science), 2001.

42. Johns B, Torres T. Costs of scaling up health interventions: a systematic review. *Health Policy and Planning*, 2005, 20:1–13.

43. *Programme of Action adopted at the International Conference on Population and Development, Cairo, 5–13 September 1994*. New York, United Nations Population Fund, 1996.

44. *United Nations Millennium Declaration*. New York, United Nations, 2000 (United Nations General Assembly Resolution A/55/2, 18 September 2000; http://www.un.org/millennium/declaration/ares552e.pdf, accessed 1 March 2006).

45. Walker J. Performance gaps, policy research, and political entrepreneurs: toward a theory of agenda setting. *Policy Studies Journal*, 1974, 3:112–116.

46. Kingdon JW. *Agendas, alternatives and public policies*. Boston, MA, and Toronto, Little, Brown and Company, 1984.

47. Doig J, Hargrove E, eds. *Leadership and innovation: a biographical perspective on entrepreneurs in government*. Baltimore and London, Johns Hopkins University Press, 1987.

48. Wilson J. *Bureaucracy: what government agencies do and why they do it*. New York, Basic Books, 1989.

49. Waddock S, Post J. Social entrepreneurs and catalytic change. *Public Administration Review*, 1991, 51:393–401.

50. Schneider M, Teske P. Toward a theory of the political entrepreneur: evidence from local government. *American Political Science Review*, 1992, 86:737–747.

51. Lovell C, Abed FH. Scaling up in health: two decades of learning in Bangladesh, In: Rohde J, Chatterjee M, Morley D, eds. *Reaching health for all*. Delhi, Oxford University Press, 1993:212–232.

52. Simmons R, Brown JW, Díaz M. Facilitating large-scale transitions to quality of care. *Studies in Family Planning*, 2002, 33:61–75.

53. National Center for the Dissemination of Disability Research (NCDDR). *A review of the literature on dissemination and knowledge utilization*. Austin, TX, Southwest Educational Development Laboratory, 1996 (http://www.ncddr.org/du/products/litreview.pdf, accessed 27 March 2006).

54. Sternin M, Sternin J, March D. Scaling up a poverty alleviation and nutrition program in Vietnam. In: Marchione TJ, ed. *Scaling up, scaling down – overcoming malnutrition in developing countries*. Amsterdam, Gordon Breach Publishers, 1999:97–118.

55. Lavis JN, Ross SE, Hurley JE et al. Examining the role of health services research in public policymaking. *The Milbank Quarterly*, 2002, 80:125–154.

56. Askew I, Matthews Z, Partridge R. *Going beyond research: a key issues paper raising discussion points related to dissemination, utilization and impact of reproductive and sexual health research*. Paper presented at: Moving Beyond Research to Influence Policy Workshop, University of Southampton, 23–24 January 2001 (http://www.socstats.soton.ac.uk/choices/workshop, accessed 14 February 2005).

57. Satia JK, Mavlankar D, Menon I. *Scaling up for child survival – key issues*. In: *Collection of concept papers, case-studies and experience-sharing: regional workshop on scaling up for child survival activities, 20–23 August 1985*. Ahmedabad, Indian Institute of Management, 1985.

58. Gladwell M. *The tipping point: how little things can make a big difference*. Boston, MA, Little, Brown and Company, 2000.

59. Walker JL. The diffusion of innovations among the American states. *The American Political Science Review*, 1969, 63:880–899.

60. Klinmahorm S, Ireland K. NGO–government collaboration in Bangkok. In: Edwards M, Hulme D, eds. *Making a difference: NGOs and development in a changing world*. London, Earthscan Publications Ltd, 1992:60–69.

61. Howes M, Sattar MG. Bigger and better? Scaling up strategies pursued by BRAC 1972–1991. In: Edwards M, Hulme D, eds. *Making a difference: NGOs and development in a changing world*. London: Earthscan Publications Ltd, 1992:99–110.

62. Díaz M, Simmons R, Díaz J et al. Action research to enhance reproductive choice in a Brazilian municipality: the Santa Barbara Project. In: Haberland N, Measham D, eds. *Responding to Cairo: case-studies of changing practice in reproductive health and family planning.* New York, The Population Council, 2002:355–375.

63. Uphoff N, Esman MJ, Krishna A. *Reasons for success: learning from instructive experiences in rural development.* West Hartford, CT, Kumarian Press, 1998.

64. Simmons R, Hall P, Díaz J et al. The strategic approach to contraceptive introduction. *Studies in Family Planning,* 1997, 28:79–94.

65. *Public expenditure management handbook.* Washington, DC, International Bank for Reconstruction and Development/World Bank, 1998.

66. Grindle MS, ed. *Politics and policy implementation in the Third World.* Princeton, NJ, Princeton University Press, 1980.

67. Migdal J, Kohli A, Shue V, eds. *State power and social forces: domination and transformation in the third world.* Cambridge, Cambridge University Press, 1994.

68. Mintrom M. Policy entrepreneurs and the diffusion of innovation. *American Journal of Political Science,* 1997, 41:738–770.

69. Buse K, Gwin C. The World Bank and global cooperation in health: the case of Bangladesh. *The Lancet,* 1998, 351:665–669.

70. Berer M. Health sector reforms: implications for sexual and reproductive health services. *Reproductive Health Matters,* 2002, 10:6–15.

71. Bossert T. Analysing the decentralization of health systems in developing countries: decision space, innovation and performance. *Social Science and Medicine,* 1998, 47:1513–1527.

72. Bossert T, Beauvais J. Decentralization of health systems in Ghana, Zambia, Uganda and the Philippines: a comparative analysis of decision space. *Health Policy and Planning,* 2002, 17:14–31.

73. Mills A, Antonius R, Danield J et al. The distribution of health planning and management responsibilities between centre and periphery: historical patterns and reform trends in four Caribbean territories. *Health Policy,* 2002, 62:65–84.

Chapter 2

Strategic choices in scaling up: introducing injectable contraception and improving quality of care in Viet Nam

Peter Fajans, Nguyen Thi Thom, Maxine Whittaker, Jay Satia,
Tran Thi Phuong Mai, Trinh Dinh Can, Do Thi Thanh Nhan, Nancy Newton[a]

Summary

This chapter analyses the process of scaling up introduction of the injectable contraceptive depot-medroxyprogesterone acetate (DMPA) as part of a package of interventions to improve quality of care in the provision of all contraceptives in the Vietnamese family planning programme. After a strategic assessment of the need for contraceptive introduction and pilot testing of the interventions in three provinces, these interventions were scaled up to 21 of Viet Nam's 64 provinces. Although DMPA was widely introduced, going to scale did not fully achieve the gains in quality of care for all methods found in the pilot phase. Three interrelated variables affected this outcome: the degree of change required in the service delivery system, the pace of expansion, and available resources to support expansion. In this case, scaling up proceeded faster than was desirable, given the extensive changes entailed by the interventions and the limitations in resources. Before embarking on rapid expansion involving complex programmatic changes, planners of scaling-up strategies should carefully assess the balance between these three variables.

---

[a] The first seven authors of this paper were all involved in the scaling-up process. At the time of project implementation Nguyen Thi Thom was a researcher at the National Committee for Population and Family Planning, involved in the strategic assessment, pilot project and scaling up as a resource person. Tran Thi Phuong Mai of the Ministry of Health was Deputy Director of the Department of Reproductive Health. Peter Fajans of the World Health Organization and Maxine Whittaker and Jay Satia, both of the International Council on the Management of Population Programmes, were members of the technical assistance team. Trinh Dinh Can was responsible for project implementation for the National Committee for Population and Family Planning. Do Thi Thanh Nhan served as the project representative from the Viet Nam Women's Union. Nancy Newton, an independent consultant, provided conceptual and editorial input.

Introduction

Introducing new contraceptive methods into health services often poses a fundamental dilemma. Provision of the new method is typically tested in a pilot setting in which a great deal of attention is paid to information for clients, counselling, and the technical and managerial aspects of service delivery. In contrast, other available contraceptive methods continue to be provided as they were before, often with inadequate quality of care. The Strategic Approach to Contraceptive Introduction,[1] sponsored by the World Health Organization (WHO), emphasizes the importance of ensuring quality of care in the provision of all available contraceptive methods when new ones are added to programmes (1). Viet Nam was one of the initial countries to implement the Strategic Approach. In the early 1990s, concerns arose about quality of care in the family planning programme in Viet Nam[2] and calls emerged for greater availability of a wider range of contraceptives (2, 3). Following a strategic assessment of the need for contraceptive introduction, a pilot project demonstrated that the injectable contraceptive depot-medroxyprogesterone acetate (DMPA) could be successfully introduced as part of a comprehensive effort to improve quality of care in the provision of all contraceptive methods.

This case-study describes the pilot project and its scaling up, showing how strategic choices influenced the extent to which success could be maintained during the process of expansion. Successful scaling up implies that key features of new practices tested and proven to be effective remain intact during expansion, because otherwise pilot results cannot be replicated. Literature on scaling up calls attention to the risk of losing the essential characteristics of interventions as they are expanded to new areas (4). This chapter chronicles how this risk was addressed in interventions designed to broaden contraceptive choice and quality of care in Viet Nam. Factors in the broader environment that influence strategic choices are highlighted as well. If programme managers understand the factors that affect scaling up, they can make decisions that increase the odds of achieving intended outcomes.

---

[1] This was the precursor of the Strategic Approach to Strengthening Reproductive Health Policies and Programmes.

[2] The Vietnamese family planning programme involves two key ministries, the National Committee for Population and Family Planning (NCPFP, now known as Viet Nam Commission for Population, Family and Children, VCPFC) and the Ministry of Health as well as several mass organizations of which the Viet Nam Women's Union (VWU) is the most active. The NCPFP is responsible for the policy, financial and logistic aspects of the programme; the Ministry of Health is responsible for service delivery through its network of facilities in 64 provinces, 653 districts and almost 11 000 commune health centres; and VWU cadres promote family planning in communities.

The Vietnamese family planning programme was driven by an explicit policy to reduce population growth and a focus on modern, highly effective, and long-acting methods (5). Information provided to clients stressed the benefits of family planning for national development and "family happiness" (6, 7). The intrauterine device (IUD) dominated the method mix, accounting for 62% of contraceptive use. Natural methods, including withdrawal, represented 25% of use; female sterilization 6%; oral contraceptives 4%, and male methods (condom and vasectomy) 3%. Use of injectable contraceptives was negligible, and they were provided only in the private sector (8). Payments and incentives given to health workers and clients for providing or accepting the IUD or female sterilization called into question the extent of informed choice and clients' ability to freely choose a contraceptive method.

In 1993, programme managers proposed introducing the injectable contraceptive DMPA and the subdermal implant Norplant® into the national programme to broaden the method mix and thereby increase contraceptive prevalence. However, previous unsuccessful efforts to introduce new contraceptive methods raised concerns. Earlier introduction of oral contraceptives, which had taken place without a specific strategy or plan, had had minimal impact. Past small-scale trials of DMPA introduction found extremely high discontinuation rates, and evaluations noted the lack of adequate counselling concerning side-effects, provider misunderstanding of side-effects and their management, and poor follow-up of clients (9–11). A small-scale trial of Norplant® introduction also identified numerous difficulties in service delivery, including providers who had not been trained in removal, limited counselling, and insufficient coordination among government, nongovernmental organizations and donor agencies (12).

In light of these unsatisfactory outcomes, senior programme managers sought a more systematic approach to contraceptive introduction. When they learned about the recently developed Strategic Approach, they were eager to test this methodology to support introduction of DMPA and Norplant®. The approach had credibility, as it was espoused by a respected group of international agencies including WHO. Its phased process consisting of three stages – a strategic assessment, testing interventions and scaling up (1, 13) – would allow the national programme to move cautiously, without making a formal commitment to complete adoption or change from the outset. It also represented a means to avoid the difficulties experienced in earlier introductory efforts.

Application of the Strategic Approach began in late 1994 with a participatory strategic assessment of the need for contraceptive introduction, carried out by the Ministry of Health, the National Committee of Population and Family Planning (NCPFP) and the Viet Nam Women's Union (VWU), with technical assistance from several international partners. At a 1995 national dissemination workshop, participants reviewed and agreed with the assessment team's conclusions, which emphasized that priority should be given to improving quality of care in the provision of already available methods and that introduction of contraceptives currently not available within the public sector should be approached with caution. After intensive discussions, senior NCPFP and Ministry of Health officials and representatives from international partner agencies agreed that Norplant® should not be introduced at that time, because the service delivery system lacked the capacity to provide it with good quality of care. However, they approved the assessment team's suggestion to develop and test a systematic strategy for introducing DMPA as part of a broader effort to strengthen quality of care (14). The government was keenly interested in developing a strategy for introducing DMPA, an interest reinforced by the arrival of 160 000 donated doses of DMPA in the national warehouse. In light of this, the assessment team felt that a pilot project focusing solely on improving quality of care, without introducing DMPA, would have been rejected by the government. At the same time, the assessment experience had produced a consensus among key programme managers concerning the importance of improving quality of care in the provision of all contraceptive methods. Therefore a pilot project was proposed which would introduce DMPA while simultaneously addressing the overall quality of care.

The pilot project

The pilot project introducing DMPA as part of a package of interventions to improve quality of care for all contraceptive methods involved both service delivery interventions and research in three provinces. In the first year, 1996, activities focused on four districts selected from three provinces. In the second year, activities expanded to eight communes in each of the four districts. A five-person central team designed and managed the introductory study, with technical support from international partners. Central team members who had been involved in the strategic assessment included representatives from the Maternal and Child Health and Family Planning Department of the Ministry of Health, the Centre for Population Studies and Information of the NCPFP, and the VWU. At the provincial level a three-person team, composed of one member each from the health sector, the Provincial Committee for Population and Family Planning and the Provincial Women's Union, coordinated activities.

The project tested a range of managerial and service delivery modifications that dealt with weaknesses found during the strategic assessment in the six dimensions of quality of care outlined by Bruce (15).[3] DMPA was introduced into health facilities to broaden contraceptive choice. Training was designed to upgrade the technical competence of health workers and family planning field motivators. Training addressed knowledge and skills in counselling and information provision to support informed choice and use of the chosen method. It also covered the management of side-effects, infection control and other related areas of reproductive health. The principles and values of quality of care and reproductive rights framed these competencies. Information, education and communication (IEC) materials that emphasized voluntary choice of methods and how to use a chosen contraceptive were developed, tested and distributed to strengthen information given to current and potential clients. These materials replaced existing ones focused on the need for smaller families and the advantages of different contraceptive methods. Increased attention was given to ensuring client privacy at health facilities. The service mix was broadened through additional training and supervision to emphasize prevention and treatment of reproductive tract infections (RTIs) as well as post-abortion care and counselling.

New management and supervisory practices were developed and introduced. Management information tools – including client-held cards for all methods and a logbook for DMPA users, which recorded management of side-effects and dates of next visits – were tested to support follow-up and continuity mechanisms. In preparation for implementing these interventions, each pilot site conducted a situational analysis and used the findings to develop procedures to improve client flow, logistics management and infection control. Supervision was reoriented from inspection and a focus on achievement of demographic objectives to helping providers and managers direct their attention to quality of care and client-responsiveness. Teams of providers and managers at service delivery points were encouraged to seek the views of their clients and the community and to respond to them through action plans and follow-up activities. This was reinforced by routine collection of data on quality-of-care indicators.

Training was a key process for introducing the interventions. The skills of master trainers from the training institute of the Ministry of Health were strengthened; these trainers then trained provincial teams, who in turn trained providers and field motivators in the prov-

---

[3] Informed choice, information giving, technical competence, client-provider relations, follow-up and an appropriate constellation of services.

inces and districts. The master training team would later be available to support expansion of interventions. Training methodologies represented a further enhancement of practice in Viet Nam. Competency-based standards and principles of adult learning, wherein facilitators drew upon participants' own experiences and used interactive techniques, were quite different from the one-way teaching styles typically in use at the time. Supervisory visits, role modelling by central team members and administrative circulars reinforced the interventions. Mid-term and end-of-pilot-project dissemination workshops offered further learning opportunities. Articles about quality of care, the Strategic Approach and DMPA service delivery, published in the internal newsletters of the three agencies, helped to inform managers and providers about the interventions being tested.

Substantial effort was devoted to furthering trust, communication and collaboration between the Ministry of Health, the NCPFP and the VWU at the senior management, provincial and district levels, reinforcing the working relationships of these institutions developed during the strategic assessment. External technical advisers facilitated workshops on vision sharing, and routine meetings of the central and provincial teams contributed to the process of strengthening working relationships.

Research conducted during the pilot project included a quantitative study of DMPA acceptability, continuation and discontinuation as well as baseline and follow-up qualitative studies of client and provider perspectives and service delivery issues. Results from the first phase of qualitative studies were used to guide modifications in the interventions, especially changes in the service mix, counselling, IEC messages and the development of refresher training (16).

Results of the pilot phase

At all sites, many women showed an interest in DMPA and some began to use the method. Providing DMPA at the more accessible commune level in the second year increased adoption and facilitated follow-up and continuation. The one-year continuation rate for DMPA use in the pilot project areas was considerably higher than the rates experienced in earlier small trials in Viet Nam. Both the continuation rate and users' experience of side-effects were similar to international results. As women learned more about the method in their communities and its availability increased, the number of women choosing DMPA grew steadily. Preliminary study results suggested improvement in many of the dimensions of quality of care in the provision of all methods.

At the mid-term review workshop in March 1997, staff of the agencies involved in the project and representatives of donor and other partner organizations came together to analyse experiences from the first year of activity. The evidence convinced central team members that this systematic approach to introduction was valuable because it resulted in higher continuation rates for DMPA and a diversification of the method mix. They also saw that it benefited women. However, managers in the Ministry and the NCPFP who had not been involved in the pilot project expressed concerns that the testing was taking too much time and questioned the need for the full package of interventions. They recommended rapidly expanding introduction of DMPA, without all the other pilot interventions and without waiting until the two-year pilot project was over. Central team members and external technical advisers did not concur: they argued that rapid expansion of DMPA introduction, without the accompanying service delivery and management interventions, would not reproduce the broader improvements in quality of care found during the first year of the pilot project.

Shortly after the mid-term review, decision-makers in the NCPFP chose to proceed with only those interventions required to introduce DMPA in 11 additional provinces (hereafter called the "DMPA-only provinces"). They adapted and applied some of the principles and practices tested in the pilot project. For example, introduction of DMPA was phased, with activities beginning at the district level in only one district in each province. Introduction was later extended to a subset of communes in those districts. Site selection took into account the capacity of the facilities, staff and supervisors to support DMPA introduction with appropriate quality of care. The training curricula, IEC materials and management tools for DMPA, developed in the pilot project, were also employed. However, the range of interventions to improve broader quality of care in the provision of other contraceptives was not replicated.

At the final pilot project dissemination workshop in August 1998, participants reviewed the evidence from the pilot phase. User perspective and service delivery studies suggested that many dimensions of quality of care in the provision of all methods improved in the pilot sites. Some aspects of infection control were better, providers' knowledge of contraceptive methods increased and provider bias diminished. Improvements were also seen in counselling, provision of information to clients and client–provider relations. For example, providers paid more attention to clients' privacy and showed greater respect for clients' wishes. Abortion clients were more likely to receive post-abortion contraception. Provincial and district programme managers, family planning motivators and community members demonstrated greater support for the concept of informed choice based on balanced information and counselling. Gaps remained, however, particularly in the quality of counselling for methods other than DMPA and for other related reproductive health services such as abortion care and the management of RTIs (*16*).

At the workshop, case-studies compared the experiences of the three pilot project provinces and the 11 DMPA-only provinces. Workshop participants concluded that the more comprehensive package of interventions tested in the pilot project yielded better results than the modifications implemented in the DMPA-only provinces. DMPA continuation was greater, the management of side-effects was better, and the quality of care in the delivery of all methods was superior. Based on this review, participants recommended that DMPA should be more widely introduced using the comprehensive intervention package. However, this introduction should proceed in a careful, phased manner within selected districts that met minimum standards regarding their capacity to provide an acceptable level of quality in service delivery. This set the stage for developing the next phase, which would be scaling up interventions tested in the pilot project.

Scaling up

Following the end-of-project workshop, an independent high-level committee appointed by the Ministry of Health further reviewed the evidence from the strategic assessment and pilot project, and recommended scaling up the principles and practices used in the pilot project. The central team prepared a proposal to introduce the comprehensive package of interventions in 21 of the 64 provinces (including the three of the pilot project) between January 1999 and June 2001. Though some individuals expressed concerns about the ambitiousness of the initial selection of 21 provinces, this large number was chosen for scaling up innovations within a period of less than two years because each had ongoing external donor support for family planning activities which resulted in both heightened interest in DMPA introduction and efforts to improve quality of care. There was an expectation that financial resources would be available to support the necessary programmatic activities.

Figure 2.1 shows the design of the scaling-up process in terms of the framework proposed by Simmons and Shiffman in Chapter 1. The innovation was the full package of interventions tested in the pilot project. The resource team consisted of the central team, with limited support from external advisers. External technical assistance was reduced to about 15% of that available in the pilot phase. In essence, the central team became the resource team – the primary source of guidance for scaling up. The user organization included the managers and staff at national, provincial, district and commune levels in the family planning programme. The scaling-up strategy involved implementing the full range of activities to support the introduction of the innovation and addressed both horizontal scaling up (replication of the innovation in provinces, districts and communes) and vertical scaling up (policy initiatives to institutionalize the innovation). Funding to support implementation at the district and commune levels came largely from ongoing international donor support to family planning activities[4] and from the regular budget of the national government.

A modular tool kit (Table 2.1) was a key component of the scaling-up strategy, serving as a guide for adapting and implementing the innovation. It included criteria for selecting sites and sample programme support materials. Consistent with the central government's practice of issuing guidelines and policy edicts to lower levels, the provinces selected for expansion were given the tool kit with the expectation that it would be closely followed, although with local adaptation. The central team then held workshops for the 21 provincial teams on how to use the tool kit. Each provincial team included representatives of the provincial health and family planning sectors and the Provincial Women's Union. Bringing together managers from these three institutions for a workshop was an unusual but constructive experience. Supervision and mentoring by the central team further supported the scaling-up process in the provinces. Because interventions in the pilot project had already been tested, the government saw scaling up as part of routine programme operations with no need for formal research and evaluation. Policy initiatives to institutionalize pilot project innovations included review and modification of national standards for all available contraceptive methods, and development and distribution of policy briefs for programme managers synthesizing lessons learned. Central team members continued to publish articles about the innovation. To develop the Vietnamese research community as a potential advocate for quality of care, the resource team organized a workshop for social scientists in the field of family planning. The objective was to strengthen their capacity to undertake studies on user perspectives and service delivery, as most previous social science research in reproductive health had focused predominantly on the demographic aspects of the population policy.

---

[4] WHO, the United Nations Population Fund (UNFPA) and Deutsche Gesellschaft für Technische Zusammenarbeit (GTZ).

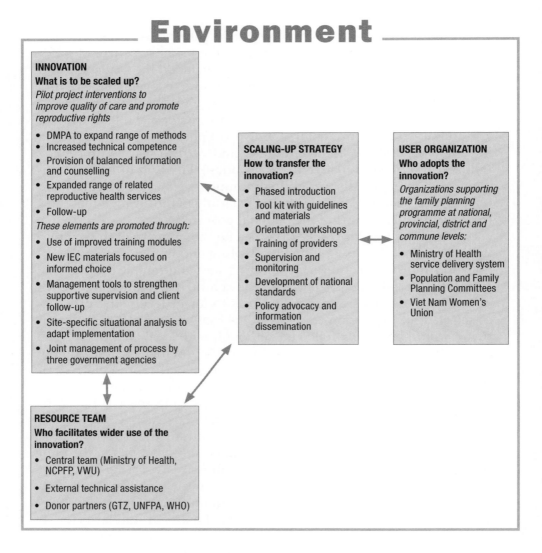

Figure 2.1 Design of the scaling-up process in Viet Nam

Outcomes of the scaling-up process

Before the pilot project, DMPA was not available in the public sector. At the end of the scaling-up phase in June 2001, about 2000 women had voluntarily adopted DMPA as their method of contraception, with a mean continuation rate of 50% at one year, similar to international experiences. Since then, scaling up of the innovation has continued as part of the government's routine programme. The NCPFP and the Ministry of Health now require provinces to submit an annual plan detailing the continuing process for DMPA introduction. The plan must include arrangements for training and logistics, assessment of the capacity of the facilities to support quality of care and other aspects detailed in the tool kit. An approved plan then receives funding from the central level, supplemented by resources from the provincial budget. By 2002, all 64 provinces had begun the process of introducing DMPA. Subsequently, it became available in half of the districts and communes in Viet Nam. In 2002, national survey data revealed that DMPA accounted for an estimated 2% of modern contraceptive method use, up from 0% in 1996. The overall method mix was also somewhat more balanced: IUD use declined to 56% (from 62% in 1993), oral contraceptive use increased to 10% (from less than 4%), and male methods (condoms and vasectomy) accounted for 9% (up from 3%) of modern method use (17).

Steps in modular tool kit for scaling up	
1. Establish task force	8. Management information systems
2. Inform stakeholders	9. Supportive supervision
3. Situational analysis and action plan	10. Community support for quality of care
4. Action plans for quality of care	11. Facility requirements for quality of care
5. Plan for training	12. Accreditation process
6. IEC for quality of care	13. Monitoring for quality of care
7. Logistics for quality of care	14. Continuous quality improvement

Each step contains information on:

▶ Rationale
▶ Methodology
▶ Illustrations of previous experience in Viet Nam
▶ Examples of materials, tools and activities
▶ Advice on adapting the materials to local conditions

Table 2.1 Contents of the modular tool kit for scaling up

Because the scaling-up process did not include a formal evaluation component, insights into the implementation and outcomes in other dimensions of quality of care come from routine service data and observations made by facilitators and central team members during supervision. Many principles and practices from the tool kit were implemented. For example, provincial and district teams used criteria in the tool kit to identify sites for scaling up. They phased the expansion process by typically choosing only two districts in each province; within each of these, they selected for start-up activities a few commune health centres that met minimum standards for quality of care. Provinces quickly adopted the logbook for DMPA users, and some used the client-held cards for all methods. Supportive supervision gained ground: provincial managers described how they discussed service implementation and problem-solving with providers, instead of looking exclusively at achievement of demographic targets. Training sessions utilized the competency-based, participatory, model training curriculum and facilitators' guides in the tool kit, and the new criteria for selection of trainers were followed. There was also evidence of an increase in client orientation. For example, some service providers asked that training and services place more emphasis on prevention and care of RTIs and HIV/AIDS, as well as on adolescent reproductive health, reflecting client and community demands. More IEC materials became available, and providers demonstrated greater understanding of the need to provide information and counselling to clients.

Despite these advances, improvement in the quality of care in provision of all contraceptive methods was less than that found during the evaluation of the pilot project. In general, training, counselling, IEC, management of side-effects, infection control and client follow-up related to DMPA provision were better than for other methods. Tool kit components were sometimes applied only to the delivery of DMPA. For example, some provincial training teams used the parts of modules that focused on this method and did not incorporate sessions that dealt with informed choice and quality of care. In some sites, IEC materials were provided for DMPA but not for other methods. Systems to monitor quality-of-care indicators were not fully implemented. The collaboration among the NCPFP, the Ministry of Health and the VWU that occurred during the pilot project was not in evidence in all provinces, and in many, the VWU was often not fully involved as a partner in scaling up. Similarly, in many districts and communes, field motivators did not receive training and thus continued to encourage long-acting contraceptives and did not engage the community in identifying needed improvements in quality of care.

Other related outcomes

Satisfied with their first experience implementing the Strategic Approach, the government decided to apply the methodology to abortion care. Following a strategic assessment in May 1997 (*18*), a pilot project to test quality-of-care interventions for comprehensive abortion care was put in place in two national hospitals, and activities are gradually being expanded to provincial hospitals. This programme gives evidence of the government's appreciation of a phased approach to introducing service delivery innovations.

The Ordinance on Population issued in 2004 demonstrates an increasing concern for quality of care in the family planning programme. This policy emphasizes the right of individuals to exercise choice of contraceptives, gives prominence to quality family planning services, counselling and improved access to information, and explicitly prohibits "preventing or forcing the utilization of family planning practices" (*19*). The recent removal of incentives formerly given to women who accepted the IUD provides further evidence of the national commitment to freedom of choice. Without a doubt, international partners and national advocates working on other initiatives have played an important part in these changes. In all likelihood, the rapid decrease in fertility among Vietnamese women – from a total fertility rate of 3.8 in 1985 to 2.2 in 2001 (*17*) – also reduced pressure on the government to pursue demographic targets and enabled the family planning programme to increase its focus on quality of care. Nevertheless, these changes represent remarkable policy shifts and significant advances for reproductive rights.

Discussion

In the course of the interventions described above, DMPA was introduced into the family planning programme in 21 provinces and its availability has since expanded to all 64 provinces. However, quality-of-care innovations related to the full range of contraceptive methods were not consistently implemented during scaling up. Reflecting on the reasons for such partial success brings to the fore three key interrelated variables that must be considered when planning and implementing strategies for scaling up: the degree of change that the innovation implies for the user organization; the pace of expansion; and the amount of resources available. Ideally, decisions about these variables are made so that there is congruence or balance among them; for example, the resources available must match the degree of change and the pace of expansion. However, these choices are often shaped by the environmental context (as depicted in Figure 2.2) and thus achieving balance may be difficult (20). As this case-study illustrates, when the three variables are out of balance, it results in trade-offs in the outcomes achieved.

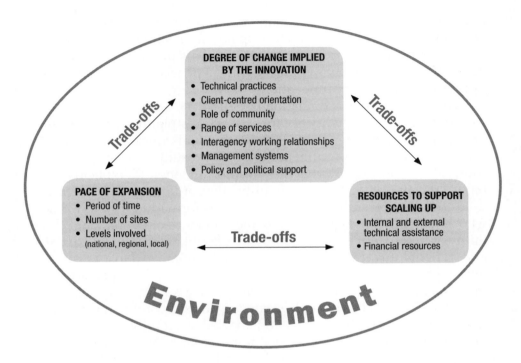

Figure 2.2 Strategic choices in scaling up: balance and trade-offs

The degree of change implied by the innovation

The innovation tested in the pilot project was a complex package of interventions aimed at improving the quality of care in family planning services. Full implementation called for much more than increasing provider knowledge and skills related to a particular technical issue: it required stronger programme and managerial capacities to support changes and a system-wide reorientation towards a client-centred approach. This new orientation involved transforming a pattern of client–provider interactions characterized by little counselling and a lack of informed choice into one of active, respectful exchanges. Providers were expected to offer balanced information, listen to clients' concerns, offer individually tailored guidance and be motivated to take the time to do so. In Viet Nam, however, prevailing beliefs among providers and managers held that women did not want a lot of information about contraceptives and choice of method was considered the domain of medical providers. Provider incentives to encourage use of long-acting methods and community mobilization to reinforce the two-child policy persisted. Information given to clients generally centred on the advantages of certain methods and the importance of family planning. A client-centred orientation called for community participation in shaping service delivery, but community voices were seen as having little relevance for what was viewed as a strictly medical concern. Thus, the new emphasis on quality of care required major programme and provider reorientation. Linking family planning services with RTI prevention and treatment and post-abortion care was a novelty in a programme focused on demographic objectives. Furthermore, the Ministry of Health, the NCPFP and the VWU were not accustomed to working in close partnership at the provincial, district and commune levels.

In contrast, the technological aspects of introducing DMPA did not demand the same degree of change. This new technology was more directly in line with the priorities of the family planning programme, which gave precedence to achieving demographic goals through increased contraceptive prevalence and use of highly effective contraceptive methods. Programme leadership had high expectations about the impact that DMPA would make on increasing contraceptive prevalence. The provision of DMPA also benefited from being a tangible, readily observable innovation, and use of the method could be measured through routine service statistics, unlike elements of quality of care such as client satisfaction and informed choice. Furthermore, injections have a strong positive cultural value for both providers and community members in Viet Nam.

In sum, the distance between the existing state of family planning services and the required change inherent in the package of interventions was large. Breaking with established norms and practices and bringing about client-centred services and policies implied a high degree of change in a family planning programme characterized by a weak capacity to provide services with good quality of care. Even in strong health systems, getting health providers to modify minor elements of routine practice is a major challenge (21).

Pace of expansion

There was a strong desire among national-level policy-makers to scale up as rapidly as possible. Family planning programme authorities in many provinces were beginning to request DMPA introduction, and national officials were eager to respond. The presence of DMPA supplies in the national warehouse reinforced this demand. In addition, members of the donor community wanted to incorporate DMPA into their projects and some were not convinced of the value of waiting for lessons to be learned from scaling up; prevailing international wisdom at the time maintained that provision of DMPA was not a complicated task. Although the resource team realized that a slower pace (scaling up initially in fewer provinces over a longer period of time) would be preferable, they felt it was more important to grasp the window of opportunity of government and donor interest in the introduction of DMPA and maintain the linkages between DMPA introduction and improvements in quality of care for all methods. In the interests of remaining engaged in the policy and programme strengthening process, scaling up proceeded at a relatively rapid pace. This strategic choice resulted in a trade-off: DMPA was made more widely available in a shorter period of time, but without all of the potential improvements in quality of care for all methods. In retrospect, and as the international literature and experience suggest, fuller replication of the package of interventions in 21 provinces might have been feasible with a more gradual process because of the extensive modifications in service delivery entailed in the innovation (Chapter 1).

Resources to support scaling up

As described earlier, resources for technical support were decreased as expansion proceeded. This choice was not a result of limited donor funding. Continuing the high degree of national ownership that had characterized the application of the Strategic Approach throughout the assessment and pilot project was considered critical for sustainable integration of the innovation into routine service delivery. At that time, the rationale held that once an innovation had been successfully tested in a pilot project, large amounts of outside support and funding would inhibit the potential for lasting change. Thus a decision was made to depend primarily on the five-person national-level resource team for provision of technical assistance and to rely on existing financial resources for implementation. In addition, the government was satisfied that the pilot project had adequately demonstrated the feasibility of implementing the package of interventions. Large-scale integration of the innovation into programme operations was considered a straightforward process.

Unexpected developments inevitably occur when working with public sector bureaucracies. Just before interventions began to be scaled up, three of the original five members of the national resource team left their positions or retired. The three new team members did not have the benefit of experience with the strategic assessment and pilot project, and the resulting understanding about the importance of interventions to improve quality of care. This reduced the resource team's capacity to support the scaling up. Moreover, the team was charged with sizeable tasks that were added to their routine work: developing and producing the tool kit, conducting orientation workshops and supervising training for 21 provinces, providing ongoing support and guidance to the process, documenting experiences and assisting in development of technical standards for all contraceptive methods.

In hindsight, the choice to decrease both the human and financial resources available to support scaling up implied a trade-off with the degree of change that could be achieved. The extensive organizational and cultural changes needed on the part of the health services were more than the resource team could support and facilitate given the rapid pace of expansion. Producing the transformation implied by the innovation, particularly at the relatively rapid pace dictated by the policy window, would have called for a massive effort on the part of a sizeable and well-equipped resource team (see Chapter 1).

Balance and trade-offs

The strategic choices made regarding any one of the three variables – the pace of expansion, resources to support scaling up, and the complexity of the innovation – affect the other two and determine the success in maintaining intact the essential features of the innovation during the process of going to scale.

The compromised decision to pursue a relatively rapid pace of expansion brought some benefit (availability of an additional contraceptive method) to more women than could have been reached with a slower pace. However, a slower pace would have had the potential to bring greater benefit (improved quality of care for all methods) to fewer people. Alternatively, the rapid pace of expansion could perhaps have been supported by a larger and more experienced resource team, which might have been able to advocate for and promote all the changes implied by the innovation. When the divergence between the nature of the innovation and the characteristics and prevailing practices of the user organization is great, full implementation of the innovation may not be possible without either a slow pace or substantial resources to facilitate its integration into routine service delivery.

Conclusion

In designing and implementing strategies for scaling up tested innovations, tensions will inevitably arise among three critical variables: the degree of change, the pace of expansion, and the resources required to achieve the desired change. Planners and implementers need to weigh the alternatives carefully and continuously reassess the implications of the trade-offs among these three variables.

Efforts to meet reproductive health needs will almost always encounter the imperative to expand innovations rapidly in order to reach the greatest number of people in the shortest possible time, given available financial resources. The potential of improved services and technologies to maximize health benefits and save lives, however, may obscure the degree of change implied by these interventions – changes in organizational culture, in managerial and technical systems, in clients and communities who need the interventions, and in the broader environment. At the same time, scaling up generally takes place in a context of constrained resources, characterized not only by limited finances but, more importantly, by weak public sector health systems with bureaucracies that are slow to adopt innovation and have few staff members to support and guide the introduction of large-scale changes.

Before undertaking to scale up innovations involving complex changes, planners and implementers would be wise to ask the following questions: What are the risks involved in moving quickly? Will a rapid pace of expansion potentially overwhelm a weak bureaucratic system? How far-reaching are the changes entailed in introducing the innovations? Are expectations so high that they are beyond existing capacities of the resource and user system? How will the capacity to manage the changes be strengthened? Is there a capacity-building plan in place and are the necessary resources committed? Is there a system to monitor and evaluate the scaling-up process? Once a set of innovations has been tested, scaling-up practitioners must reflect upon the relative risks and benefits of a more rapid versus a slower process, given the resources available to support expansion.

Although trade-offs may be unavoidable, discerning and understanding the multiple environmental factors that can affect the success of scaling up is equally important when making choices that seek to balance the degree of change implied by the innovation, the pace of expansion, and the amount of resources to support the change.

The case-study from Viet Nam provides a useful illustration of the importance of achieving an appropriate balance among the three key variables. Given the environmental circumstances that mandated a rapid pace of expansion and the large degree of change represented by the innovations tested in the pilot phase, there was a need for much greater human and financial resources to be devoted to support the development of the institutional capacity. In hindsight, the challenges of making major changes in how programmes are implemented and – even more important – changing the attitudes and practices of individual providers were greater than the resources devoted to the task. Although much was achieved in Viet Nam, the experience shows how critical it is to devote sufficient resources to building institutional capacity to support the process of scaling up an innovation. The lessons learned can help guide future efforts to scale up innovative pilot projects serving the reproductive health needs of people in Viet Nam and elsewhere.

Acknowledgements

We wish to thank the many individuals, who participated in the various activities described in this paper, for their valuable contributions. We also acknowledge funding for the implementation of the Strategic Approach in Viet Nam from the Department of Reproductive Health and Research, WHO, together with the UNFPA and GTZ offices in Hanoi.

References

1. Simmons R, Hall P, Díaz J et al. The strategic approach to contraceptive introduction. *Studies in Family Planning*, 1997, 28:79–94.

2. Jain S, Kornfield R, LeComite J et al. *Thematic evaluation: quality of family planning services in Viet Nam*. Hanoi, United Nations Population Fund, 1993.

3. Knodel J, Phan Thuc Anh, Dao Xuan Vinh. *Viet Nam's population and family planning program as viewed by its implementers*. Bangkok, The Population Council, 1995 (Population Council Regional Working Papers, South and East Asia, No. 2).

4. Korten DC, Klauss R, eds. *People-centered development: contributions toward theory and planning frameworks*. West Hartford, CT, Kumarian Press, 1984.

5. *Annex to the report to the National Meeting for Mid-term Review and Implementation of the Strategy of Population and Family Planning Programme to the year 2000, Hanoi, 11–13 November 1993*. Hanoi, National Committee for Population and Family Planning and General Statistical Office, 1993.

6. Vu Quy Nhân. Family planning programme in Viet Nam. *Viet Nam Social Sciences*, 1994, 1:3–20.

7. Goodkind D. Viet Nam's one or two child policy in action. *Population and Development Review*, 1995, 21:85–111.

8.   *Population and family planning strategy to the year 2000.* Hanoi, National Committee for Population and Family Planning, 1993.

9.   Do Duy Che, Le Hoang Duong, Tran Thi Vinh et al. *Report on survey using contraceptive Depo Provera injection in Nam Ha Province 1992–1995.* Phu Ly, Ha Nam, 1995 (unpublished).

10. Duong Thi Cuong, Nguyen Thi My Huong. *Research on safety, effectiveness and acceptability of DMPA injectable contraceptives on Vietnamese women.* Hanoi, Institute for the Protection of Mother and New Born, 1995 (unpublished).

11. Tran Van Dong, Do Ngoc Tan. *Evaluation of safety, effectiveness and acceptability of DMPA contraception in Hai Hung Province, Viet Nam, 1995* (unpublished).

12. *Retrospective study of the Norplant trials in Viet Nam.* Hanoi, The Population Council, 1997.

13. *The Strategic Approach to Improving Reproductive Health Policies and Programmes: a summary of experiences.* Geneva, World Health Organization, 2002 (WHO/RHR/02.12).

14. Do Trong Hieu, Pham Thuy Nga, Nguyen Kim Tong et al. *An assessment of the need for contraceptive introduction in Viet Nam.* Geneva, World Health Organization, 1995 (WHO/HRP/ITT/95.3).

15. Bruce J. Fundamental elements of the quality of care: a simple framework. *Studies in Family Planning,* 1990, 21:61–91.

16. Nguyen Thi Thom, Do Trong Hieu, Vu Quy Nhân et al. The strategic approach to the introduction of DMPA as an opportunity to improve quality of care for all contraceptive methods in Viet Nam. *Asia-Pacific Population Journal,* 2000, 15:63–86.

17. *Annual survey of demographic and family planning change.* Hanoi, National Statistical Office and National Committee for Population and Family Planning, 2002.

18. Do Trong Hieu, Pham Thuy Nga, Do Phuong Mai et al. *Abortion in Viet Nam: an assessment of policy, programme and research issues.* Geneva, World Health Organization, 1999 (WHO/RHR/HRP/ITT/99.2).

19. Viet Nam Commission for Population, Family and Children (VCPFC). Ordinance on Population. *Population, Family and Children,* 2004, January–February:1–15.

20. Paul S. *Managing development programs: the lessons of success.* Boulder, CO, Westview Press, 1982.

21. Bero LA, Grilli R, Grimshaw JM et al. Closing the gap between research and practice: an overview of systematic reviews of interventions to promote the implementation of research findings. *BMJ*, 1998, 317:465–468.

Chapter 3

Quality of care in China: from pilot project to national programme

Joan Kaufman[a]*, Zhang Erli*[b]*, Xie Zhenming*[c]

Summary

China's family planning programme ranks as history's most intensive effort to control national population growth. While some have lauded China's effort to limit births as a fundamental part of its sustainable development goals, the population policy has also generated much international criticism. A long-overdue reform has begun to focus the family planning programme on client needs, informed choice of contraceptives, and better quality services. Partly inspired by the International Conference on Population and Development in 1994, the reform began as a pilot project in six counties and is now a blueprint for reorienting the national family planning programme. This chapter reviews the process by which a small innovative pilot project was scaled up into a national reform effort and the lessons learned about scaling up sensitive but needed innovation in a difficult political environment. These lessons relate to the importance of local ownership, adapting concepts to make them locally meaningful, careful choice of pilot sites to ensure success, mobilizing political networks, cultivating and educating allies in senior leadership positions, strategic use of donor funding and technical assistance, and the willingness to transfer project management to the next generation of leaders.

[a] Joan Kaufman is Director, AIDS Public Policy Project, John F. Kennedy School of Government, Harvard University; and Senior Scientist, Heller School of Social Policy and Management, Brandeis University. She was the China-based Ford Foundation Reproductive Health Programme Officer who began financial support for the Quality-of-Care Pilot Project in 1996 and worked closely with the project team on strategy and planning.

[b] Zhang Erli is former Director-General of the Statistics and Planning Department, National Population and Family Planning Commission, China. He was the pilot project's creator and the first project director; he has retained his role as senior strategist of the programme since its inception.

[c] Xie Zhenming is Deputy Director, China Population and Development Research Centre (CPDRC, previously the China Population Information and Research Center). He was a key member of the resource team and has, since 1999, directed the operational office of the Quality-of-Care Pilot Project.

Introduction

China's family planning programme ranks as history's strongest effort to curtail national population growth through deliberate birth control. While some advocates for global population control have praised China's effort to limit births as a basic part of its sustainable development goals, the population policy has also generated much criticism from governments and groups concerned about human rights. The one-child policy, introduced in 1980, aimed to encourage one birth per couple with detailed regulations and birth targets.[1] This policy has been blamed for motivating coercive measures, especially forced sterilizations and abortions, enforced by local officials on an unwilling population. From 1995, a reform of the family planning programme began to introduce a focus on individual couples' needs, informed choice of contraceptives, and better quality services. Partly inspired by the International Conference on Population and Development (ICPD), held in Cairo in 1994 (1), the reform began as a pilot project in six counties and is now a model for reorienting the national family planning programme. This chapter reviews the process by which this innovative experiment was scaled up into a national reform effort. The authors were deeply involved in the pilot project and its scaling up.

China began a concerted family planning effort in the early 1970s (2). By the end of the decade, China's national total fertility rate had dropped from nearly seven births per woman to 2.7 (3). As it was recognized that demographic momentum would fuel population growth for decades to come, the one-child policy was introduced to dramatically slow down the rate of growth.

Policy implementation was based on parity-driven prescriptions of reliable contraceptive use: an intrauterine device (IUD) after the first birth and sterilization after the second. Prior to the ICPD, there was little appreciation of clients' perspectives and quality of care. The need to protect voluntarism in couples' choice about the number and spacing of children was considered less important than achieving overall fertility goals. There was no counselling about choice of methods and medical follow-up was minimal (4). Women were obliged to accept the IUD or sterilization soon after childbirth, and those with an IUD were required to obtain regular ultrasound check-ups to confirm that the device was in place and that they were not pregnant. Couples were required to obtain official permission from local birth planning

---

[1] Birth targets refers to the number of allowed births in a given year that are set at national, provincial, and prefectural levels and are then communicated to county governments to become a basis for cadre evaluation for promotion. Regulations refer to the explicit rules on pregnancies and births, for example on who is allowed to have a second birth.

officials for allowed pregnancies and births, based on detailed regulations. Out-of-plan pregnancies had to be aborted and intense pressure, psychological and sometimes physical, was put on couples unwilling to conform.

From the start, the policy – especially the heavy-handed methods of implementing unwanted abortions and sterilizations – met with popular resistance by rural couples. Unlike their urban counterparts, rural couples have no pensions or social security; they rely on grown sons, who traditionally care for aged parents and do not marry out into other families as daughters do. Together with the persistence of Confucian traditions of son preference, the prospect of an only daughter was untenable.

China's family planning programme is managed as a top-down process, from national level to province, prefecture, county, township and, finally, village. National guidelines, regulations concerning births, population targets, monitoring and evaluation systems and standards of care are formulated at the top, by the National Population and Family Planning Commission (NPFPC) (its name was changed from State Family Planning Commission in 2003). Provinces then enact regulations and, because population control is a key national policy, all levels of government are required to provide adequate funding to local family planning bureaux to carry out the policy. In the 1980s, family planning and health services were separated, and independent family planning clinics were established at county and township levels (5).

Beginnings of reform: 1990–1995

A number of events in the first half of the 1990s contributed to the initiation of a pilot project that led to the national family planning reform. In 1991, a project aimed at introducing new contraceptive technologies to China initiated the introduction of quality improvements in family planning services, especially the concept of informed choice of contraceptive methods (6, 7). Other collaborations during the 1990s, involving the International Planned Parenthood Federation (IPPF), its affiliate the China Family Planning Association, the World Health Organization (WHO) and Chinese family planning research institutes, further developed concepts of counselling, client rights and informed choice. Nevertheless, these efforts remained uncoordinated and isolated, and there was little rethinking at the State Family Planning Commission (SFPC) about reforming the mechanisms of implementing the family planning programme.

From 1994 to 1995, a large contingent of Chinese family planning officials and researchers attended ICPD preparatory meetings in Bali, the ICPD in Cairo, and the Beijing Women's Conference, where concepts of reproductive rights and ethical perspectives on family planning programmes were discussed and widely endorsed. Following these conferences, a leading Chinese demographer translated and published a book of key documents from the meeting, including the Programme of Action and the seminal article by Judith Bruce (8) on the need for quality-of-care improvements in family planning programmes (9). The book was distributed to senior family planning policy-makers, many of whom had attended the ICPD or had previously been involved in donor-supported projects.

The senior SFPC official responsible for setting and monitoring implementation of population targets[2] participated in the ICPD and was strongly influenced by the humanism of the Bruce framework. This exposure, together with his own difficult experience in implementing population targets, made him receptive to rethinking the methods of implementing China's family planning programme. After years of trying to correct falsification of family planning data by local officials worried about performance evaluations, and observing changes resulting from the move to a market economy, the Bruce framework provided him with an appealing new approach. He believed that as market reforms advanced, client expectations for good quality services grew, especially in more economically developed areas (10). He felt that the programme had to adjust to this shift and start giving individuals greater choice in their selection of contraceptive methods and begin providing other reproductive health services. Together with like-minded colleagues from the China Population and Information Research Center (CPIRC), he formulated the idea of a pilot project in six counties to introduce quality-of-care improvements in the programme.

The goal of the proposed project was to test whether realigning the programme to people's interests and needs was possible, desirable, and would not result in additional births. All of the project initiators supported the government's population control goals in principle, but they had misgivings about the way the policy had been implemented and felt that serious reform was necessary. Their vision was supported by the Minister of Family Planning, who provided them with an opportunity to try out this radical new approach that could potentially question the underpinnings of a top-down mandated birth control policy. Many years of dialogue between the SFPC and the United Nations Population Fund (UNFPA) on the issue of voluntarism in the family planning programme may have helped to create some of the pressure for change and to influence the Minister's thinking.

---

[2] Zhang Erli, the second author of this paper.

In 1995, the Minister made an official call for "two reorientations" of the Chinese family planning programme: to move the programme away from family planning alone and integrate it closely with economic and social development and address population issues in a comprehensive manner; and to shift programme implementation from primary reliance on social constraints, such as coercion and fines, to gradually institutionalizing interest-driven methods, such as individual choice and demand-based services, along with coordinated information, education and communication (IEC), comprehensive services and scientific management (11). The early proposal by the Minister promoted the idea of keeping a tight control on population, but doing so without coercive measures. The two reorientations were to be achieved nationally by 2010, along with other goals of the government's ninth Five-Year Plan (1996–2001). The Minister saw the pilot project as an opportunity to move the two reorientations forward (12).

The Quality-of-Care Pilot Project, Phase 1: 1995–1999

Initiation in six counties: 1995–1997

The Quality-of-Care Pilot Project was initiated in 1995 as an experiment to test out the new approach called for in the two reorientations. During the early years, project innovators were isolated and relied on the Minister for their political support. Local participation was not mandated by the SFPC. The project initiators stipulated in advance that no central or provincial government funds would be provided to carry out project activities. The intention of this was to demonstrate sustainability and to ensure local commitment. The project leaders selected counties where they had good personal relationships with lower-level managers in the family planning system. Five rural counties and one city in six provinces on China's eastern seaboard (Jiangsu, Jilin, Liaoning, Shandong, Shanghai and Zhejiang) were chosen to participate. Their social and economic development had rapidly progressed since the beginning of the economic reforms in the late 1970s. Total fertility rates in these counties were under two; thus there was little fear that introducing the new approach would result in a surge of births.

The main objective of the project was to introduce the six elements of quality of care developed by Bruce (8) into family planning services in the six counties.[3] Project leaders supported the counties with training, materials and regular workshops to share experience.

---

[3] The six elements of quality of care are: informed choice, information giving, technical competence, client-provider relations, follow-up and an appropriate constellation of services (8).

In the early years, the project can be described as a context-specific quality-of-care approach, which retained China's population control imperatives but relaxed some of its restrictions, especially in the area of contraceptive choice. The project implemented a more human-centred programme with greater levels of informed choice, counselling and follow-up for side-effects. The counties began to offer couples a choice of five contraceptive methods (IUDs, oral contraceptives, condoms, Norplant© implants and sterilization), provided more face-to-face counselling and computer-based information about contraceptive methods, and increased the constellation of services for women, all within the context of strict regulations about the number of allowed births. While all counties followed common guidelines for improving service quality based on the six elements of quality of care (8), there were some differences in emphasis. For example, one county focused on developing youth services, another on improvements in counselling and IEC activities, and another on informed choice.

At the end of 1996, project leaders sought and received funding from the Ford Foundation to begin a process of evaluating the impact of their effort to improve the quality of services. This began with a workshop where the six counties proposed indicators for evaluating their quality-of-care improvements and international participants presented the quality-of-care experience from other countries. After one year of the project, with no observable increase in birth rates, a meeting was held between the Minister and the mayors of the six pilot counties, together with their provincial and county family planning directors in which the mayors and directors endorsed the project and convinced the Minister that the reorientation should continue and expand.

Expansion: 1997–1999

Reassured that the pilot project was not jeopardizing fertility goals, the Minister agreed to expand the project to five new counties at the end of 1997. This modest official expansion involved replication and little change in approach, because the main goal until then had been to achieve support for expansion. However, as the project and the Minister's decision to expand it became known within provinces, many other counties perceived this as a "green light" to visit pilot sites to learn more and to begin some level of similar activities in their own counties, without formal project involvement. They were eager to join an initiative where some of the policy restrictions on parity-specific method requirements were being relaxed.

From 1997 to 1999 a second track of quality-of-care innovations began, characterized by rapid replication of the pilot county experience by neighbouring counties within some of the same provinces (Jiangsu,

Shandong, Zhejiang) and endorsed by the Minister. By 1998, over 200 counties (of about 3000 counties in 31 provinces in the country) were participating informally, using their own resources. These informal county participants were invited to attend project-sponsored training courses on different topics, with occasional participation by international quality-of-care consultants. These second-track counties can be classified as spontaneous expansion, where innovations from the original pilots were adopted with some local adaptations. The number of second-track counties expanded rapidly, especially in the provinces where the pilot counties were located, reaching over 800 by early 2000.

A number of activities helped to consolidate learning and reshape the programme to conform more closely to international concepts of quality of care. Continued Ford Foundation support in 1998, which included international technical assistance, helped project leaders evaluate their efforts to introduce international practices and to develop strategies for training and other activities. Eight senior officials from the SFPC visited India in 1998 to meet government counterparts and researchers to learn about India's experience in lifting demographic targets, moving towards a reproductive health approach and using new indicators to evaluate the programme. Those who participated in the study tour to India became important internal advocates for project expansion within the SFPC. A contact group, comprising the project leaders and core international partners, was formed in 1998 to provide strategic direction for the project. This group played an important role for several years, supporting and informing internal debates about strategy and expansion.

In late 1998, a crisis and an opportunity helped to push the Quality-of-Care Pilot Project closer to centre stage. A leadership transition occurred and the project initiators, with help from external facilitators, succeeded in developing a strategy to ensure continuity and ongoing political support. The Minister was changing, and the project's creator and chief strategist retired from his official SFPC post and was thus obliged to step aside as director. Project management was transferred to the SFPC's new Director General of the Science and Technology Division – an important development for the potential expansion of quality innovations within the national family planning service network and the SFPC. The project's creator recognized the need to have the new director learn about the project who soon recognized its value. Similarly, the Vice-Minister responsible for the programme was cultivated and became an advocate for reform. The new director began consolidation of donor-supported projects to sustain the reform effort and, with her backing and collaboration, the core team set up an operational office at CPIRC from where they maintained day-to-day management of activities. The project creator continued his involvement as a consultant and volunteer, though without an official role. With great benefit to the project, ownership had passed to powerful new insiders in the government with the ear of the new Minister.

At the International Symposium on Quality of Care, held in Beijing in November 1999, both the new Minister and the Vice-Minister gave speeches endorsing the reform (13, 14). Following that meeting, the contact group discussed plans for project expansion, based on the findings of the qualitative assessment undertaken the previous year. An influential national advisory board was set up for the project during the symposium. This board included researchers, provincial family planning officials, women's activists and representatives of nongovernmental organizations (NGOs) involved in reproductive health research and projects, who provided both validity and increased advocacy for the project.

Evaluation of the initial pilots

Evaluation research involved an assessment of the original six counties using an adaptation of the Strategic Approach to Strengthening Reproductive Health Policies and Programmes (15, 16). An international researcher involved in the development of the Strategic Approach participated in the research. The assessment was carried out in 1998 by an interdisciplinary team of more than 20 Chinese and two international participants, including researchers, project team staff and programme managers. Several members of the Quality-of-Care Pilot Project national advisory board participated in the evaluation. The direct involvement of advisory board members further broadened the base of support for the project and helped to publicize it.

The assessment team interviewed programme managers, service providers, local leaders and community members, with special emphasis on married women of reproductive age. The study showed many positive changes. Stable low fertility was maintained and women enjoyed greater freedom in choosing a contraceptive method and relations between clients and providers had improved, as had those between family planning programme managers and the local population. Women reported that they felt more respected and cared for, and local leaders indicated that tensions were eased in implementing the family planning programme. The full report was published in Chinese in 1999 (16). An in-depth analysis of one of the original pilot counties revealed some changes in the contraceptive method mix accompanying the introduction of informed choice, especially in moving away from sterilizations and towards condoms (17). These method mix changes are important indications of the move away from government-dictated method use based on parity. A study undertaken among 2000 women in one of the second-track counties showed that, as the quality-of-care index increased over three years, abortions decreased significantly (18).

These studies indicate that even though this first phase of the project only offered a limited version of the international quality-of-care model proposed by Bruce, progress was made in beginning to improve clients' choice of method and in reducing contraceptive failures. The project counties adapted the quality-of-care approach to local realities, including, especially, the requirements of China's population policy that contraception must be used. The main achievement during Phase 1 was improving the method mix, especially by providing alternative choices to sterilization, though there was little change in the pressure to abort out-of-plan births. Many pilot counties reported that abortion numbers decreased as contraceptive choice and follow-up increased, which was attributed to fewer contraceptive failures (19). More importantly, the project began to introduce concepts of client orientation in services, and the focus shifted from top-down implementation to more client-need driven and more user-friendly services.

The Quality-of-Care Pilot Project, Phase 2: 2000–2004

The second phase of the project included geographical expansion and functional diversification and the beginning of institutionalization within the SFPC. Responding to the growing interest in the approach from an increasing number of counties, the project was expanded from 11 to 19 counties. Activities were diversified to include new services and approaches as well as management changes. Four new subprojects were initiated, including: further development of informed choice within the Chinese context; improvement of the family planning management information system to incorporate indicators and approaches to measure quality of services; further work on incorporating prevention, treatment and diagnosis of reproductive tract infections (RTIs) into routine family planning services; and expansion of the project to the less developed western regions of the country. The subproject on improvement of the family planning management information system produced new indicators on quality of care that were disseminated for national use in 2002. The project leadership selected influential national universities and research institutions to lead and manage the work, distributing ownership to powerful allies and away from exclusive SFPC control. Respected national and international experts were brought in as consultants, thereby further broadening the base of support for the project among academics and related institutions already working on reproductive health.

Of the four subprojects, the western expansion was critical for demonstrating the potential to scale up the project nationally. Unlike the coastal counties, where social and economic development was advanced and total fertility rates were below two, fertility desires were higher in the poorer western regions. If the reform could be implemented in these counties without extra resources and without raising fertility, then senior leadership would endorse its expansion on a larger scale.

In February 2000, the western subproject was initiated in six counties, all committed to undertaking the reforms without extra funding. These counties faced more economic difficulty and more limited personnel capacity than the pilot counties in the east. Recognizing this, the project team permitted them to begin by adding services that were relatively easy to implement and/or met immediate needs, such as RTI check-ups or other women's health improvements including infertility treatments. As in the eastern pilots in Phase 1, the western pilots were allowed to move gradually to a pattern of greater informed choice. Self-designed project activities gave the counties a strong sense of ownership.

The Quality-of-Care Pilot Project as a model for national reform

By the end of 2000, the momentum of reform was evident and ownership of the effort by SFPC's senior leaders was clear. This momentum was enhanced by another major initiative promoting quality of care: the UNFPA 32-county reproductive health improvement project. The UNFPA effort was nationally designed and standardized with extensive donor input. It sought to improve reproductive health in rural counties that were more diverse, and in some cases poorer, than those involved in the Quality-of-Care Pilot Project. The project provided opportunities for training, the development of new counselling and IEC materials and technical assistance on evaluation and monitoring. It supported a re-thinking of programme goals, methods and evaluation criteria and promoted a wider reproductive health agenda.

Consensus at the top levels of leadership was reflected in a series of official documents enshrining the concept of informed choice of contraceptives and emphasizing the necessity of protecting the rights of citizens and safeguarding them from coercion in the implementation of the family planning programme. Donor inputs were increasingly being coordinated by the SFPC to support its national reform effort, rather than handled as separate programmes within different parts of the Commission. This institutionalization ties together a number of similar efforts that began around the same time as the Quality-of-Care Pilot Project. Several donor-initiated projects promoted many of the same ICPD themes: reproductive health and rights, informed choice, better quality services and client orientation. These other projects, involving UNFPA, the IPPF and several United States NGOs, were originally developed and carried out in isolation from the Quality-of-Care Pilot Project, but have now begun to come together. The project provided an acceptable local model for consolidating these various post-ICPD donor programmes that had not previously been seen as workable in the China context.

In the second half of the 1990s, several departments in the SFPC had also introduced reform-oriented initiatives, such as formulating a new population law, an IEC campaign emphasizing gender equity in family life, improving the female child survival environment, and distributing new technical guidelines. By 2000 the SFPC began to bring these initiatives together with the Quality-of-Care Pilot Project. The SFPC began to refer to the more than 800 second-track counties as "the SFPC quality counties" or the "provincial pilots", thereby officially beginning to claim ownership of the experiment. In an important meeting in northern China in 2000, the new Minister held a television conference with all the directors of provincial family planning commissions, in which he endorsed the quality-of-care approach.

In December 2000, a "white paper" issued by the central government, entitled *China's population and development in the 21st century*, endorsed the changes, albeit within a continued emphasis on population control (*20*). This important document used the language of the two reorientations and explicitly stated that quality services should be provided (Article 14) and that citizens' legal rights should be protected in the implementation of the family planning programme. This document was followed in early 2001 by new regulations for technical service management in family planning for all family planning workers and government officials, promoting quality services and informed choice of methods. In mid-2001, a draft Population Law was submitted to the National People's Congress with provisions for criminal prosecution of cadres who use coercion to implement family planning and reiterating the language on informed choice (*21*). The Law was passed and became effective in December 2002.

In 2001, some of China's leading women's activists were involved in an activity intended to help family planning staff to see the programme through women's eyes and to increase gender sensitivity in programme implementation. Training used participatory methodologies and approaches developed by the IPPF/Western Hemisphere Region, in collaboration with the Latin American and Caribbean Women's Health Network (22). For the first time, Chinese women activists from the All China Women's Federation, university-based women's studies centres and women's NGOs were willing to engage with the family planning programme, after years of silent opposition to rights abuses within it.

The SFPC launched a new effort in 2002 to establish 100 "quality advanced counties", representing every province (two to three counties per province), from which to model province-wide expansions. These counties were selected from those involved in the Quality-of-Care Pilot Project, from UNFPA's project counties and from the second-track quality pilots. The 33 criteria and standards to evaluate quality services in these counties are based on indicators developed in the second phase of the Quality-of-Care Pilot Project.

A further expansion of the project was developed during 2003 and was launched in early 2004. This expansion includes diversification through new subprojects and geographical expansion to new sites. Diversification is responding to newly identified challenges, such as HIV/AIDS training and services for rural migrants living in urban areas, in line with new pro-poor government welfare policies and with the growing HIV/AIDS epidemic. The NPFPC is increasingly coordinating all donor funding and technical assistance to support its national reform effort. At an important project training workshop in early 2004, new evaluation standards developed by the project were presented, including six indicators used to measure "the people's satisfaction rate".

Lessons learned about scaling up

The Chinese Quality-of-Care Pilot Project experience and its success to date in scaling up offers important lessons about how to move controversial innovations to a national stage in a sensitive political environment. Many of these lessons provide additional support for insights derived from other scaling-up literature.

1. Foster government ownership

The Quality-of-Care Pilot Project was devised and initiated from within the SFPC and was not donor-driven. In China, a major mechanism of institutional change is the use of pilot demonstration projects. Model areas are often held up for national replication, and testing ideas is always considered more relevant than wholesale application of ideas from abroad. The still limited role of NGOs in mobilizing change and the central role of powerful officials, constrained by Communist Party mandates that discourage true experimentation from going forward, make the China context somewhat different from other regions. A major challenge for scaling up in China is to build innovation from within the government, which remains the main actor in service delivery and policy formulation. NGOs can play a role in demonstrating innovative approaches, but without government ownership and endorsement they are unlikely to lead to national reform.

When the momentum of reform and SFPC's senior leaders' endorsement were evident by the end of 2000, the effort moved rapidly to deliberate scaling up and institutionalization, with a clear focus on organizational change (23). The political support and increasing ownership by SFPC's senior leaders helped to move the pilot project to the second phase, from a replicated demonstration project to an expanded and functionally diversified project, and shortly thereafter toward institutionalization within the national family planning programme.

2. Choose pilots carefully to ensure success and local ownership

Although the project leaders utilized a long tradition in China of model counties to garner support for the reforms, they altered their approach in several significant ways. They provided no additional funding so as to demonstrate sustainability and to attract local enthusiasts, who would willingly navigate the potential difficulties of the new approach. Participating counties volunteered knowing that they would receive no additional funds to carry out project activities. Counties were carefully chosen to reassure senior leaders that there would not be any adverse fertility outcomes of the reform. Starting small, and choosing their original project sites strategically to ensure success, allowed project leaders to make a case for expansion. They carefully built a movement for change from the bottom up, by allowing other interested counties to participate freely in training and workshops and encouraging them to visit pilot sites.

The Chinese scaling-up experience shares common features with other international projects, especially ones undertaken by governments rather than NGOs. Initial scaling up involved replication as a way to expand the pilot experiences to other counties. Staged replication as conceptualized by Wazir & Van Oudenhoven (24) involves a process of pilot testing, followed by carefully evaluated implementation in different sites and then expansion more broadly. Demand from below and careful pilot testing and replication, though locally adapted and owned, was a central feature of the China experience.

3. Cultivate powerful allies and be willing to transfer project management to new leaders

A number of strategies were used by the project team to consolidate gains in Phase 1 and encourage further expansion. Attracting the attention of the senior SFPC leadership expanded the base of support. These efforts to foster ownership of the project by a widening circle of leaders who assumed positions of power under the new Minister built an internal constituency for reform. The willingness of the project creator to step aside and transfer the strategic management of the project to a more appropriate location ensured its integration into the technical work of the SFPC. The creation of an operational office outside the SFPC guaranteed that the work moved forward during these transitions.

4. Use research and technical assistance to define expansion needs

Research during Phase 1 was used to generate evidence on project achievements and to guide the reform effort. The project management team then used the research findings to orchestrate the development of four new subprojects, in order to develop the systems and mechanisms for integration of quality of care into the day-to-day operations of the national family planning programme. International technical assistance and funding contributed to the credibility and visibility of the research effort and findings. Research and technical assistance have continued to guide the evolution of the Quality-of-Care Pilot Project during its second phase.

5. Adapt concepts to make them locally meaningful

The Quality-of-Care Pilot Project was based on adoption of a new international paradigm agreed to at the ICPD, which spoke to recognized problems in the China context. The quality-of-care concepts were adapted considerably to fit national realities, and then even more to fit local needs and opportunities. Adaptation was especially needed to fit the constrained environment for free and informed choice and the restrictions on couples' ability to make decisions regarding the number of children and the spacing of births. Such adaptation made it possible for the paradigm shift to occur within a political setting that is resistant to change.

The project leaders were all innovative public sector bureaucratic actors who used their positions of leadership and opportunities for internal advocacy to drive the reform. Their clear messages were relevant to the local areas, especially because of the credibility of the messengers. They used personal contacts to advance the quality-of-care agenda and strategically mobilized technical assistance and donor funding both to gain legitimacy and to increase internal visibility. In other words, the project innovators applied many of the strategies that the literature suggests are important in effective scaling up: they recognized policy windows and cultivated ownership for the experiment among their leaders, recognized and encouraged demand for the reforms from lower levels, and carried out the reforms using phased implementation, adaptation and learning (23, Chapter 1).

Conclusion

Quality-of-care reform in China is still a work in progress. Although significant improvements have been achieved, many challenges remain. As the reform effort expands, there is a continuing need for further clarification and application of international concepts in the China context. Although the concept of informed choice of contraceptive methods has moved far beyond its initial limited interpretation in the early 1990s, it is still not truly implemented as intended by the ICPD, that is, as a programme that prioritizes reproductive rights over population goals and guarantees full voluntarism in the timing and numbers of births. Women in the pilot counties are still not permitted to decline contraceptive use or to choose freely the number and spacing of their children. Although they have more choice in selecting their contraceptive methods and more freedom to change them, they are still urged to abort out-of-plan births. The family planning programme still has a long way to go in terms of adopting a gender perspective in its design and implementation.

Many mechanisms still remain to ensure that contraceptives are being used and to discourage out-of-plan births. There are numerous financial and administrative burdens on couples to ensure that they comply with population goals, such as registering for permission to become pregnant and give birth. Incremental gains are being made, however, through the quality-of-care reform to push back some policy restrictions on birth spacing and the requirement to register for the first birth. Overall, the reform is changing the interface between the family planning programme and the population and instilling an appreciation among local managers and service providers for user perspectives and for client rights to good quality services, information and reasonable policies. Introducing the concept of informed choice through a bottom-up process of change is building pressure for greater voluntarism in the family planning programme and is helping to support reformers at the national level who seek to back away from target-driven, coercive and restrictive aspects of population planning (17). However, the programme requires systematic external evaluation to document real changes in informed choice and contraceptive method mix, so as to respond to the concerns of sceptics and critics.

That the Quality-of-Care Pilot Project is home-grown is probably the major reason for its success in taking the reform as far as it has come. In the sensitive area of China's family planning programme, no experiment or reform effort imposed by external actors could garner the political support necessary to go forward. The project team educated and cultivated senior leaders and broadened their base of support with the SFPC and the provincial-level governments and family planning commissions, capitalizing on other programmes under way to support their agenda and vision for change. Subprojects were strategically distributed to be led by influential national organizations. Despite uncertainties about commitment and understanding of the project by a new generation of SFPC leaders, the project creators recognized the need to transfer ownership of the experiment to a new group of power brokers who could take the project to the national stage. Recognizing the value of the project, the new director used her influence and considerable insights to scale it up as the centrepiece of a national reform effort. In fact, her recognition in 1999 that the project would not succeed unless integrated with the other work of the SFPC gave the project its most crucial advocate within the government and set the stage for the major scaling up that ensued. She actively pushed for coordination of the project with other donor-supported reform efforts at the same time as spearheading the incorporation of these reforms into the national programme. The vision stemmed from a group of internal reformers with a humanistic perspective and immediate practical problems to solve. They used a window of opportunity to begin a long-overdue reform to one of the world's most controversial programmes.

Acknowledgements

We acknowledge the contributions of Gu Baochang and Zhao Baige, who have been central actors in the Quality-of-Care Pilot Project and larger programme reforms. We would also like to acknowledge the substantial contributions of the University of Michigan, International Council on Management of Population Programmes (ICOMP), and the Population Council in providing technical assistance to the project since 1995, especially Ruth Simmons and Jay Satia. We are grateful to the Ford Foundation for financial support since 1997. Achievements are mainly due to the many provincial, prefectural and county actors involved in the project since 1995 from all the pilot counties, as well as the subproject directors and the national and international consultants.

References

1. *Programme of Action adopted at the International Conference on Population and Development, Cairo, 5–13 September 1994.* New York, United Nations Population Fund, 1996.

2. Tien HY. Wan, Xi, Shao: how China meets its population problem. *International Family Planning Perspectives*, 1980, 6:65–73.

3. Banister J. *China's changing population*. Stanford, CA, Stanford University Press, 1987.

4. Kaufman J, Zhang ZR, Qiao XJ et al. Quality of family planning services in rural China. *Studies in Family Planning*, 1992, 23:73–84.

5. Kaufman J, Zhang ZR, Qiao XJ et al. The creation of family planning service stations in China. *International Family Planning Perspectives*, 1992, 18:18–23.

6. Tu P. A study of the introduction of new contraceptives and improvement of service quality in rural China [in Chinese]. *Population and Family Planning*, 1995, 6:43–48.

7. Tu P, Qiu S, Fang H et al. Acceptance, efficacy, and side-effects of Norplant© implants in four counties in North China. *Studies in Family Planning*, 1997, 28:122–131.

8. Bruce J. Fundamental elements of quality of care: a simple framework. *Studies in Family Planning*, 1990, 21:61–91.

9. Gu B. *Reproductive health and family planning: international perspectives and approaches [in Chinese]*. Beijing, China Population Press, 1996.

10. Zhang E. *From a number-centred officer to a quality-of-care advocator: a personal story*. Paper presented at: Asia Pacific Conference on Reproductive Health, Manila, 15–18 February 2001.

11. Peng P. Address to: National Symposium on Exchanges of Experiences of "Three Integrations" in Family Planning [in Chinese]. In: *China Family Planning Yearbook 1996. Beijing, China Family Planning Yearbook Editorial Committee, 1996.*

12. Gu B, Zhang E, Xie Z. Toward a quality of care approach: reorientation of the family planning programme in China. *Innovations: Institutionalizing Reproductive Health Programmes*, ICOMP, 1999, 7–8:39–52.

13. Zhang W. *China's population and family planning programme in the 21st century*. Presentation at: International Conference on Quality of Care, Beijing, 6 June 2000.

14. *Report on the International Symposium on Quality of Care in China, Beijing, 17–19 November 1999*. New York, The Population Council, 2000.

15. Simmons R, Hall P, Díaz J et al. The strategic approach to contraceptive introduction. *Studies in Family Planning*, 1997, 28:79–94.

16. Zhang E, Gu B, Xie Z, eds. *The first phase Quality-of-Care Pilot Project situational evaluation report, 1995–1998* [in Chinese]. Beijing, China Population Press, 1999.

17. Gu B, Simmons R, Szatkowski D. Offering a choice of contraceptives in Deqing County, China: changing practice in the family planning program since 1995. In: Haberland N, Measham D, eds. *Responding to Cairo: case-studies of changing practice in reproductive health and family planning*. New York, The Population Council, 2002:58–73.

18. Li Y, Dong G, Yue H et al. The influence of quality of care on the acceptability of contraceptive methods in Jiangsu, China. *China Journal of Family Planning*, 1999, 7:54–57.

19. Gu B. *Reorienting China's family planning program: an experiment on quality of care since 1995*. Paper presented at: Annual meeting of the Population Association of America, Los Angeles, CA, 23–25 March 2000.

20. *China's population and development in the 21st century*. Beijing, State Council of the People's Republic of China, Information Office, 2000 (white paper).

21. Winckler E. Chinese reproductive policy at the turn of the millennium: dynamic stability. *Population and Development Review*, 2002, 28:379–418.

22. *Manual to evaluate quality of care from a gender perspective*. New York, International Planned Parenthood Federation/Western Hemisphere Region, Inc., 2000.

23. Simmons R, Brown J, Díaz M. Facilitating large-scale transitions to quality of care: an idea whose time has come. *Studies in Family Planning*, 2002, 33:61–75.

24. Wazir R, Van Oudenhoven N. *Increasing the coverage of social programmes*. Paris, United Nations Educational, Scientific and Cultural Organization, 1998.

Chapter 4

Expanding contraceptive choice and improving quality of care in Zambia's Copperbelt: moving from pilot projects to regional programmes

John P. Skibiak[a], Peter Mijere[b], Mary Zama[c]

Summary

This case-study explores the programmatic challenges of moving from pilot interventions to regional programmes. It documents the history of an initiative to scale up reproductive health interventions, developed and tested between 1996 and 2000 in Zambia's Copperbelt Province. The interventions included an expansion of the range of contraceptive methods available at health facilities, the development of innovative training approaches for health-care workers, and the testing of strategies to reach out to communities. This chapter highlights the challenges facing programme designers as they must decide which elements of a pilot study to scale up, the structures most appropriate for managing the process, and the pace and breadth of the expansion effort. Finally, it provides a conceptual framework to guide the scaling-up process and to weigh the potential trade-offs between increasing scale and the need to maintain quality, local values, local relevance and sustainability.

[a] John Skibiak, an anthropologist, was Director of the Population Council's Expanding Contraceptive Choice (ECC) programme in Africa. He was a member of the Zambia Contraceptive Needs Assessment team in 1995 and technical adviser to the ECC Pilot Study and Pilots to Regional Programmes (PRP) initiative described in this study.

[b] Peter Mijere is a public health physician and Deputy Chief of Party for SHARE, a USAID-funded initiative to address HIV/AIDS in Zambia. During his tenure as Director of the Copperbelt Provincial Office (2000–2004) he had management responsibility for the PRP initiative.

[c] Mary Zama, a public health nurse, is Consultant to the Population Council. She was Project Manager of the ECC Pilot Study from 1996 to 2001 and continued in that position throughout the PRP initiative. She resides in the Copperbelt and continues to manage a host of interventions designed to expand contraceptive choice and improve quality of care.

Introduction

Pilots to Regional Programmes (PRP) is the name of a broad-based initiative for bringing to scale a series of reproductive health interventions, which had been developed and tested between 1996 and 2000 in Zambia's Copperbelt Province. Launched in 2002, PRP aims to expand contraceptive choice and increase the availability of quality reproductive health services, especially family planning, in all eight of the Copperbelt's rural and peri-urban districts. It also seeks to field-test a model for scaling up reproductive health interventions, originally implemented on a pilot basis. The model employs a three-phased process in which districts adhere to a common set of quality standards while maintaining the flexibility to decide, based on local needs and conditions, the most appropriate means of achieving these standards and the relative investment they intend to make in doing so.

This case-study explores the programmatic challenges of moving from pilot study to broad-based initiative. It documents the history of the initiative, more specifically the circumstances leading to its development, the scaling up of activities and its achievements. It also describes a conceptual framework that guided the scaling-up process, while at the same time weighing the potential trade-offs between increasing scale and the need to maintain quality, local values, local relevance and sustainability.

From strategic assessment to pilot study

In 1995, the Zambia Ministry of Health sponsored a strategic assessment of contraceptive needs, applying a methodology outlined in the Strategic Approach to Strengthening Reproductive Health Policies and Programmes developed by the World Health Organization (WHO).[1] Supported by WHO and the Population Council, the assessment proved pivotal in shaping the future of reproductive health services in Zambia (2). It identified key health policy concerns, provided a framework for research on contraceptive introduction, and served as a catalyst for the development of Zambia's first family planning service delivery guidelines. It also influenced the procurement of new contraceptive methods and the phasing-out of others, such as high-dose oral contraceptives.

Based on the assessment's recommendations, a number of pilot studies were eventually carried out, each of which sought to strength-

---

[1] The WHO Strategic Approach is a systematic, three-stage approach for identifying and prioritizing reproductive health-care needs, for testing practical solutions to those needs and for bringing to scale the successes, taking account of the lessons learned (1).

en the availability of new and/or underutilized methods, while at the same time using the introduction of those methods as a means to improve the quality of services in general. The largest and by far most ambitious of these studies took place between 1996 and 2000 among selected health centres in three newly created rural health districts of the Copperbelt Province. The impetus behind the study was twofold: first there was the low utilization of contraception, and second was the dramatic imbalance in the composition of Zambia's limited method mix. In 1995, contraceptive prevalence of modern methods was only 7%, with half of all users opting for the pill, and the other half relying primarily on the intrauterine device (IUD) and sterilization (2). The explanation had to do with the weak public sector service delivery system, poor provider competence, limited access to services by large segments of the population, and – in contrast to its neighbouring countries – the virtual absence of any injectable contraceptive in the public sector.

For many years, depot-medroxyprogesterone acetate (DMPA) was a popular method among Zambia's family planning users. By the early 1980s, however, reports of its abuse in neighbouring Zimbabwe (previously Rhodesia) sparked calls for its removal from public sector services. Derided within the Zambian medical establishment, and blamed for side-effects for which there was no medical basis, DMPA was soon withdrawn from the national contraceptive method mix.

On field visits conducted during the 1995 strategic assessment, demand for the long-acting injectable was still widespread, particularly among rural women for whom the burdens of contraceptive resupply were particularly heavy. At the time, other contraceptive methods were frequently out of stock, and the existing logistics system did not supply facilities with sufficient stocks to allow advance distribution of oral contraceptives on any meaningful scale. The biases against DMPA, however, also remained strong. Many senior Ministry of Health staff had been providers when DMPA was withdrawn and still felt the impact of their exposure to the negative publicity. Field-based staff, by contrast, exhibited far fewer biases and many of them felt it was important to reintroduce the product.

The assessment concluded that fundamental changes were needed in the provision of reproductive health services and especially in the composition of Zambia's method mix. In part, this meant a reintroduction of DMPA. Even more critical was the need to broaden method choice overall. Although the range of methods theoretically available to public sector clients was broad, the weak service delivery system meant that few rural facilities ever had more than one or two methods in stock. On the rare occasion where more methods were available, poor provider training meant that staff were often unfamiliar with them or, in the case of brands of oral contraceptives, their different formulations.

The assessment's recommendations found a receptive audience. Within one year, the Ministry of Health and CARE International, a nongovernmental organization, had agreed to conduct a pilot study that would enhance contraceptive choice in three newly created districts of the Copperbelt Province. Technical support for the development and implementation of the project was provided by WHO and the Population Council. In April 1996, the pilot study got under way. Employing a quasi-experimental research design with 11 experimental and 10 control health centres, the study tested the effectiveness of new service delivery and training strategies, as well as the introduction of new contraceptives.

The years of the pilot study were a tumultuous period for Zambia's public sector health-care system, as implementation of the national health reforms had begun in earnest. The reforms embodied many features now common to health reforms worldwide, including decentralization and greater autonomy for the regions, and increased efforts at cost recovery. However, a distinctive feature of the Zambian model was the transfer of all service delivery responsibilities from the Ministry of Health to a newly formed Central Board of Health, and the reclassification of all public sector providers from permanent civil-servant status to limited-term contractors.

By obliging health personnel to reapply for their own positions, the reform process created uncertainty throughout all levels of the health system. Policy-makers were unclear about the direction the reforms were taking and were unwilling to commit either human or financial resources to new programmes or projects. Equally affected were the providers, whose lack of job security undermined efforts to strengthen services, introduce new training programmes, or engage in potentially sensitive activities such as introducing injectables – or even showing support for such a move.

The process of reform severely affected the pilot study. Turnover, especially among trained staff, was extremely high. By the end of the project's second year, only about a third of its 20 or so trained providers were still active. The reform process also undermined the study's strategy to use evidence to change attitudes and policy. Although key reproductive health managers in Lusaka routinely received project data and visited participating districts, they were often hesitant to forward their observations to senior administrators with the power to change policy. Like their counterparts at the service delivery level, managers were understandably reluctant to stand out or challenge the status quo. Ultimately, such fears led to a hiatus in project activities of over a year.

Four years after it began, the pilot study formally ended. Findings were presented at a two-day dissemination workshop in Ndola, capital of the Copperbelt Province, which was attended by more than 60 participants, including four members of the original strategic assessment team (3). Data from service statistics, an internal mid-term evaluation, feedback from the three participating health districts, and pre- and post-intervention situation analyses left little doubt that the study had had major impact on the scope and quantity of services at the 11 participating health centres. Under the leadership of a project manager, contracted by the Ministry of Health, the pilot project had trained health-care personnel in the provision of family planning services; it had provided more specialized training in IUD insertion and the screening and treatment of sexually transmitted infections (STIs), improved counselling tools and strengthened providers' counselling skills. It had also established referral systems; introduced three new contraceptives – DMPA, the female condom and emergency contraception; and furnished the centres with new supplies and equipment.

The project also employed a variety of media to communicate its accomplishments. For example, it introduced a local newsletter, which highlighted the contributions of all health facility staff – from providers, to messengers, to management. It also successfully mobilized villages to play an active role in the delivery and management of reproductive health services, seeking out the support of local opinion leaders and working through the mechanism of the local chief's tours.

At the service delivery level, the impact of study interventions was also evident. Data collected by CARE indicated substantial increases in contraceptive usage as well as a significant broadening of the overall method mix. In the 24 months following the start-up of field-based interventions, for example, the average number of new contraceptive users per quarter (480) was over twice that of the quarter prior to the study intervention (220). Finally, the study saw improvements in quality of care, as measured by baseline and end-of-project situation analyses (4).

After two days of discussion, the dissemination workshop recommended that the study's interventions be scaled up throughout all eight of the Copperbelt's rural and peri-urban health districts. Participants also provided direction as to how the effort should take place. They suggested, for example, that the equipment, supplies and even personnel involved in the pilot study should not be absorbed into routine operations of the Central Board of Health, but should rather be reserved for the scaling-up effort. They also recommended that the

new contraceptive methods introduced by the pilot study be distributed through the public sector logistics system. Finally, workshop participants called on the Ministry of Health to formally recognize the
important role of DMPA within the method mix and support its full
incorporation into the service delivery system. Within one month, the
Central Board of Health approved these recommendations and gave
a green light to scale up efforts to enhance contraceptive choice and
improve quality of care throughout the Copperbelt.

A conceptual framework for scaling up

In the months following the dissemination workshop, the team
responsible for drafting the intervention plan – the project manager
of the Copperbelt study, the director of the Copperbelt Provincial
Health Office, and a technical adviser from the Population Council –
found themselves grappling with a host of operational issues. On one
hand, they recognized that scaling up would imply a massive undertaking: the number of service delivery points, for example, would increase almost fivefold from 11 to at least 48, while the population of
the districts covered would jump from 238 000 to roughly a million. At
the same time, they acknowledged that key aspects of the scaling-up
process remained unclear: Which activities would be scaled up? Who
would do what? And how and when would the scaling up take place?

As the team grappled with possible answers to these concerns, they
gradually came to realize that these three issues were not just isolated
sets of problems, but were interrelated and in fact encompassed the
central programmatic issues and challenges associated with scaling
up in general. This realization led the team to adopt these concerns as
the main axes of a simple, yet ultimately effective framework to guide
the design of the scaling-up process. The framework, illustrated in
Figure 4.1, is represented as a triangle, with each point corresponding to one of the three key concerns: the *content* of intervention activities (what is to be scaled up?); the *process*, that is the breadth of scaling
up over time and place (where and when would it be done?); and the
organizational implications of scaling up (who would do what and how,
and by what mechanisms?). These constituent parts of the framework
are discussed on the following pages.

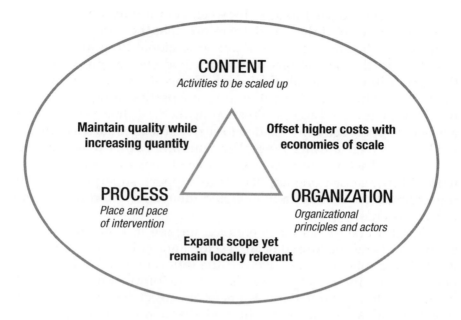

Figure 4.1 A conceptual framework for scaling up pilot interventions

Content

The literature on large-scale transitions to quality of care highlights the dangers of piecemeal approaches to scaling up, because they often sacrifice the integrity and cohesion of the intervention for the sake of operational expedience (Chapter 1). At the same time there is a need to simplify complex interventions to help facilitate their sustainable scaling up. In many pilot initiatives, the range of potentially replicable interventions can be immense. In the Copperbelt pilot study, for example, numerous activities were undertaken and tested; yet nowhere was there evidence to suggest that the study's success depended on the presence of each one. A dilemma facing any design team, therefore, is in deciding what – out of the vast experience of a pilot study – makes the most sense to introduce or expand. In the conceptual framework shown in Figure 4.1, this question is addressed by the dimension of content.

In the case of the Copperbelt pilot study, the design team reviewed the existing data, consulted extensively with district planners and providers, and concluded that the study's success rested not on any single intervention but on a combination of the study's three main focus areas: broadened method choice, improved technical competence of providers and strengthened linkages between community and the health sector. It was around these foci, therefore, that the design team chose to structure the content of the Pilots to Regional Programmes (PRP) initiative. In the case of broadening method choice, efforts involved the establishment of a minimal method mix – a set of contraceptive methods to which any client attending any participating health centre would be guaranteed access.[2] Broadening method choice also included a host of support activities needed to sustain the mix, such as functioning logistics mechanisms, referral systems and outreach mechanisms.

A second set of activities was intended to ensure provider competence. This included ongoing technical support, supervision and the implementation of both traditional and innovative self-directed training approaches.

The third set of activities entailed forging linkages between the community and the formal health sector, and within the health sector itself. These interventions involved the innovative use of local chiefs and other traditional leaders to disseminate information about reproductive health; the active involvement of project staff in community-based sensitization meetings; the revitalization of community-based health associations or "neighbourhoods", safe motherhood committees and "circles of friends"; and the publication of newsletters to share the experiences of health-care providers.

Process

The second dimension of the conceptual framework relates to the spatial and temporal aspects of the scaling-up effort. These include both the geographical scope of the intervention as well as the timing or pace of implementation.

The selection of health facilities to launch the scaling-up process was no easy task. The districts (and facilities within them) were markedly diverse with respect to their degree of urbanization, population size and density, level of health-care services and contraceptive prevalence. They were also diverse with respect to their exposure to the content of the interventions, as three of the eight districts contained health centres that had already participated in the initial pilot study. The playing field, therefore, did not start out even, and the political implications of some districts benefiting more than others figured prominently in the design process.

---

[2] Under the PRP initiative, the minimal method mix includes male and female condoms, a dedicated emergency contraceptive pill or combined oral contraceptives repackaged for emergency contraception use, the intrauterine device CuT380, DMPA, both a combined and a progesterone only contraceptive pill, bilateral tubal ligation and the Standard Days Method.

On the issue of timing, several possibilities presented themselves. Would scaling up start in the three original districts, expand to facilities never reached during the pilot, and then gradually move out to encompass facilities in the remaining five districts? Or would it begin by giving all eight districts an initial equal taste of what the project had to offer? Ultimately, considerations over content and timing converged. PRP would begin simultaneously in all eight districts, but the approach would be gradual, starting with a series of targeted interventions in at least two service delivery sites (designated as centres of excellence) per district and achieving district-wide coverage by the end of the initiative.

Implementation progressed through three distinct phases of varying lengths. During the first phase, which averaged about 18 months, 21 centres of excellence implemented a basic package of interventions. The package included the introduction of a common set of contraceptive methods and services, the application of innovative training strategies and the establishment of new community-based initiatives. The primary goal of this phase was to guarantee minimum standards of quality of care at each centre of excellence, so that they could serve as demonstration sites that could expose the other facilities to the full range of activities.

The second phase of the scaling-up effort entailed a process of reflection and analysis, culminating in the formulation of district-specific implementation plans. Over a period of about three months, each district set out its long-term goals with respect to the three content areas: contraceptive choice, provider competence and community linkages. This strategy ensured that each district only scaled up what made sense to them, and that each package of interventions reflected the unique characteristics of the district in which it was being implemented. This tailoring was seen as an indispensable element in balancing the inherent tension between the growth in the number of participating service delivery sites and the level of resources required to ensure the quality of the intervention.

During the third phase, which again lasted approximately 18 months, the bulk of the initiative's resources were used to help districts implement their plans, using the centres of excellence as springboards to expand interventions to neighbouring health-care facilities and communities.

Organization

The third dimension of the conceptual framework involved the organization of the scaling-up effort. How was scaling up to be done, by whom, and by what mechanisms?

Implementation of activities under the pilot study was carried out by two organizations, CARE International and the Zambia Central Board of Health. Both agencies followed a single protocol, but the responsibilities and funding sources of each were distinct. Their involvement was coordinated from Lusaka, where the headquarters of both were situated. As the design team turned its attention to organizing and managing a province-wide intervention, it soon became evident that the top-down, parallel structure of the pilot study would no longer be appropriate. Scaling up demanded more coordinated funding and management. It required strengthened communication and local transport, and it needed mechanisms to ensure that the interventions reflected the different needs and capabilities of the districts where scaling up would occur. Considering economies of scale also took on far greater importance. These factors pointed towards stronger horizontal linkages among districts, greater local ownership and a consolidation of management roles and responsibilities.

In responding to these needs, the design team proposed a new organizational structure that would be fully integrated with existing public sector services at both the provincial and district levels. Under this arrangement, management responsibility for the initiative fell to the Director of the Copperbelt Provincial Health Office and a team of technical advisers, led by the former project manager of the pilot study. Working hand in hand with coordinators designated by each participating health district, the advisers helped design and support activities in each of the three content areas: expanding contraceptive choice, training and the establishment of community outreach. From the start, programme implementation became a collaborative effort between the province, which provided technical and financial support, and the districts as the local coordinating and implementing agencies. Over time, however, the role of the Provincial Health Office diminished as districts gradually assumed responsibility for the content and pace of the scaling-up process. From the reflection and analysis phase onwards, it was the districts that determined which interventions would be expanded and how the expansion would take place. As districts recognized the advantages of reducing costs and maximizing economies of scale, they began to take control of management decisions, pool resources and share expenses. The Provincial Health Office did continue providing technical and financial support, but the organizational structure of PRP became less centralized.

Resolving tensions of the scaling-up process

Since its launch in 2002, the Pilots to Regional Programmes initiative has earned itself the reputation as being an innovative and cost-effective programme for scaling up high-quality family planning services in rural and peri-urban areas of Zambia. It has been the subject of rigorous observation and widespread dissemination, both nationally and regionally, and it has played a pivotal role in the introduction of new contraceptive technologies, including the formal registration in 2005 of the injectable contraceptive DMPA with the Zambia Drug and Poisons Board (5). Contraceptive prevalence in the Copperbelt's eight districts is now among the highest in rural Zambia, with many women having access to methods and services typically available only in urban settings. PRP's ability to respond to regional differences and local needs has prompted requests by the Central Board of Health and the donor community to scale up to national coverage. How, then, can this success be explained? How did use of the conceptual framework guiding the development of scaling-up strategies contribute to the success of the initiative?

Internal tensions are, to some degree, inherent in any scaling-up effort. The project design team found that the interrelationships between each point of the framework offered a practical entry point for relieving many of these tensions, thereby minimizing their impact at the outset. The inverse relationship between quality and quantity (or scale), for example, is one linkage the design team found could be addressed through interventions relating to content and process. Similarly, the dimensions of content and organization provided ample opportunities to maximize efficiencies and thereby minimize the higher costs of moving to scale. Finally, the relationship between process and organization highlighted the trade-offs between broadening geographical coverage and maintaining responsiveness to local needs and circumstances.

The conceptual framework rendered these conflicts more manageable and provided the team with a practical tool for making sense of the ambiguities associated with moving from pilots to regional programmes. How this was achieved is explained below.

Quality versus quantity: linking content and process

In moving to scale, the notions of quality and quantity are often at odds. As output increases – be it of services, clients or trained staff – the input required to sustain it should in relative terms decline, but it is precisely that decline in inputs (with its associated efficiencies and cost-savings) that can threaten the attributes that made the pilot intervention(s) so successful in the first place (6). PRP's response was to strike a balance between the two extremes – to maximize economies of scale while at the same time preserving the attributes of local control and management. It achieved this balance by exposing districts to a common set of strategies for addressing the three focus areas, but then allowing them to adapt the content of those strategies and to pace themselves with respect to their implementation. Key interventions across the three focus areas were built on common foundations and principles, but the precise timing and content of those interventions depended on decisions taken at the district level.

One of the best examples of this interface between content and process was the phased application of PRP's two training programmes for providers: a traditional classroom approach for training of trainers, and an on-site self-directed learning programme that enabled providers to follow a more flexible, independent course of readings and exercises, closely supervised by routine visits from district and/or project staff. Technically, both programmes offered equally effective and equally comprehensive instruction in the delivery of reproductive health services. Programmatically, though, their greatest strength lay in their adaptability to the constraints and realities of ever-evolving social and environmental contexts. Under the self-directed programme, for example, the cost per trainee was less than half that of the classroom alternative, but the self-directed programme was far more time consuming and was also dependent on adequate access to transport by district supervisors, something that not all districts could provide equally well. The classroom approach, in contrast, offered speed and efficiency, but it also meant removing providers from their local health facilities, which rural districts (and even many urban ones) with health posts staffed by one or two persons cannot easily afford to do.

The phased intervention process worked by exposing all the districts to the two broad training regimens, and then by providing them with the authority to decide what made most sense locally and the flexibility to pace themselves – to apply the right strategy at the right time. As services at health facilities were scaled up, the demand for trained staff increased. At no time, however, did that demand force districts to compromise quality of the training effort by implementing cost-saving measures such as: pushing the limits of classroom size, reducing the face-to-face interaction between instructors and trainees, following a single PRP-wide training schedule, or implementing approaches they could not afford. Instead, the ability of districts to pace themselves and to choose the format of their training activities meant that they were able to respond appropriately to local variations in staff attrition, service expansion and resource availability. At any given point in time, someone in some district was being trained, either on site or centrally. Within the first two years of the project, the districts had successfully trained 120 formal sector service providers – six times the number trained during the entire life of the initial pilot study – 41 of whom were trained under the self-directed programme and 79 in formal classroom settings. More specialized trainings were also conducted, particularly to increase access to IUDs. In addition, the districts hired and trained 205 community-based distributors and over 500 community-based counsellors of the Standard Days Method. By retaining control of the process and determining when training was appropriate, the districts trained more people than ever before, but on a scale that was manageable and appropriate to their needs, without ever compromising the quality or integrity of the training itself.

Maximizing economies of scale: linking content and organization

Scaling up always implies a tenuous balance between the increase in inputs needed to expand activities and the level of benefits expected. In the previous section, managing this trade-off entailed both the application of different interventions and the delegation of authority to apply those interventions in ways that best suited the needs of each district. The focus in that instance was very much on local autonomy and the realities of that locality. The imbalance between inputs and outputs can also be corrected effectively through greater integration, specifically by exploiting the potential synergies that exist across districts. By maximizing economies of scale and realizing the efficiencies that come from such scale, districts can vary the content of their programmes without undermining either their integrity or quality.

One notable example of such synergies was in the area of contraceptive choice. As noted earlier, the cornerstone of expanded choice under PRP was the right of every health facility client to have access to a minimal mix of contraceptive methods, either directly at the service delivery point or through an efficient referral system. Although all districts agreed to offer such a minimal mix, they recognized that no single approach would apply to all. Dedicated or even repackaged emergency contraception pills were not initially available in Zambia, female condoms were in short supply, and the provision of long-term methods such as injectables and IUDs had always been especially problematic at smaller facilities. For many districts, therefore, filling these gaps would have implied overwhelming investments in time and resources.

The strategy to synchronize content and achieve economies of scale operated at two levels. At one level, it allowed districts to achieve the critical mass necessary to justify large-scale production or even procurement of needed goods and services. One example of this was emergency contraception. The absence of a dedicated product undermined PRP's ability to ensure quality contraception services. Therefore, the decision was taken early on to repackage combined oral contraceptives for emergency contraception. Though widely practised throughout the world, the repackaging effort in Zambia was, from the start, a highly complex, labour-intensive endeavour. It involved the large-scale procurement of commodities from central Ministry of Health stores, along with the authorization to repackage them from the national Drug and Poisons Boards. It required letters of support from international agencies and entailed the production of appropriate packaging consistent with national requirements. Finally, it involved the repackaging of the commodities themselves. The effort required to produce a repackaged emergency contraception pill was substantial and would not have been justified by the demand generated by just one or two individual districts. It was made possible by strong central management at the provincial level, and by the fact that the production levels needed to make the effort worthwhile were commensurate with the demand for the product by all eight districts.

Maximizing economies of scale also proved highly effective in dealing with resource disparities horizontally across the Copperbelt's eight districts – disparities that in many cases affected the districts' ability to provide certain contraceptive options. One approach involved a cost-saving scheme that rewarded districts for contributing to the broader implementation of PRP interventions. The contributions could be in kind, such as food and refreshments during provider trainings, or fuel and vehicle use for supervision, or they could include the services of skilled personnel for training, supervision or service delivery. In return, districts received a credit, which they could then redeem for resources from recipient districts, or for supplemental financial support to undertake activities related to broadening method choice, strengthening technical competence, or enhancing community outreach.

Though simple in theory, implementation of the credit scheme proved challenging, especially the formulation of formal exchange mechanisms. However, it moved forward, in large part because of strong interdistrict collaboration and ongoing support from the project manager. The scheme did, for example, prompt certain districts, particularly those in peri-urban areas, to provide IUD insertions on a mobile basis and train providers from neighbouring districts. In other instances, referral fees were eliminated at urban hospitals in exchange for greater efforts to meet client needs at rural tertiary facilities. In some cases, hospital staff even began outreach activities, offering more advanced technical skills to meet the needs of their rural neighbours.

The strengthening of interdistrict linkages also made it possible to maximize economies of scale by encouraging districts to pool assets and exchange material resources such as transport, training facilities, equipment and supplies. By the second year of the initiative, the districts were conducting joint training; they were collectively procuring equipment, supplies and commodities and collaborating on other activities, such as annual planning, that they once pursued on their own. They also introduced a series of exchange programmes, whereby staff from one district served as external observers and examiners in the training programmes of another. In short, the organizational structure facilitated the expansion effort and, in the process, increased efficiency by reducing duplication. Now all districts are providing more clients with more methods than ever before. The number of new contraceptive users at participating health centres, for example, has risen steadily from approximately 1000 per quarter to current levels of almost 3000. The expansion has taken place within the context of diverse service delivery schemes, tailored to meet the unique conditions of each district, with some relying more heavily on referrals and others providing a wider range of methods on site.

Remaining locally relevant in the midst of expansion: linking organization and process

The move to scale is often characterized by the tendency to formalize and standardize roles, responsibilities and procedures (see Chapter 2). In some ways, the trend is paradoxical, for as systems are being formalized, the environments within which they operate typically become more diverse and complex. Whether it is more people, more districts or more municipalities, there is always the risk that the interventions become less appropriate for the diverse contexts in which they will be applied. A major challenge of the scaling-up process, therefore, was to ensure that expansion did not occur at the expense of relevance or local ownership.

Under the initial pilot study, a host of interventions were introduced to encourage communities to adopt a more active role in the management of health sector interventions and to increase awareness of reproductive health risks. Many of these, such as chief's tours, community discussions and outreach services, have already been mentioned. Though the designers of PRP drew heavily on the experience of these interventions, they also recognized that these activities alone could not guarantee ownership of PRP or even buy-in on the part of those communities affected by it. To make the content of PRP as meaningful and relevant as possible, therefore, the pace of the intervention process was tied to the evolving management responsibilities of the participating districts – in other words, to the dimension of organization. As the districts assumed greater control over the direction and management of activities – particularly after the formal handover of decision-making authority in phase two of the scaling-up process – they were empowered and encouraged to tailor interventions to reflect local needs, implementation capacities and interests.

The devolution of management responsibilities was facilitated both by the phased implementation process and by a number of activities focused on the third content area, community linkages. One such activity was the decentralization of information. Building on the experience of the earlier pilot study, PRP reintroduced in 2002 an illustrated newsletter that brought to life many of the initiative's major accomplishments and findings. Geared to front-line health-care workers, the newsletter nevertheless circulated widely among planners and decision-makers at all levels of the health-care system. The dissemination of information also relied on face-to-face contact. At various points during the life of the study, meetings were held to disseminate research findings, particularly the results of surveys and evaluation activities.

A second strategy to encourage local control over the implementation process was to ensure the involvement of key community members, including traditional authorities and other cultural leaders. In some communities, local chiefs were mobilized to support PRP initiatives and advocate for behaviour change. In others, technical staff helped traditional counsellors to incorporate reproductive health messages in their counselling of young women at key rites of passage associated with menarche and marriage. Finally, PRP capitalized on the dominant role of men in both community and domestic life by involving them as health agents and spokesmen for programme initiatives. This was especially successful in the promotion of the Standard Days Method.

As a result of these interventions, communities are today exercising a more direct role in shaping the kinds of health services available to them. Chiefs and other local leaders, for example, have actively lobbied districts to extend the operating hours of local clinics – they have even called for the replacement of poorly performing health personnel. Local development committees are also exerting more direct influence over the day-to-day operations of their health facilities. Some, in fact, were instrumental in ensuring that certain contraceptive options, such as natural family planning, were made available locally. Even at the individual level, community members now report that PRP's emphasis on choice has demonstrated to them the importance of this factor, and has given them the confidence to demand choice in all aspects of health care.

Conclusion

The greatest challenges in scaling up reside in the practical, organizational transformation of a small pilot study to a broad-based programmatic intervention. It was the resolution of strategic choices concerning content, process and organization that forced those planning the PRP initiative to come to grips with such issues as scale, context, organization and sustainability. And it was the design of effective strategies that yielded the results and successes described in the previous pages.

Now all eight of the Copperbelt's rural and peri-urban districts have in place organizational mechanisms for supporting PRP interventions that are fully integrated into their existing operational structures and sustained financially by the province and districts themselves. The Zambia Ministry of Health has formally identified the PRP initiative as a best practice in reproductive health and has selected its framework as the model for scaling up reproductive health services over the coming decade. The Ministry has also requested assistance from the Population Council and WHO to develop funding proposals that will make such an expansion possible.

However, the sustainability of PRP will not depend on the province alone or on the enthusiasm of the Ministry of Health. The national health system itself is once again undergoing major reforms – reforms that even include the abolition of the Central Board of Health. The Copperbelt, too, is undergoing social and economic change as reopened mines breathe life into once economically depressed areas and once active areas slide into decline. The end of funding to PRP from the United States Agency for International Development (USAID), which occurred in August 2005, is testing the initiative's sustainability, the depth of its local ownership and the degree of public sector confidence in its ability to scale up reproductive health services. Whether the participating districts and provinces can sustain their commitment to the activities of PRP remains to be seen. There can be little doubt, however, that the conceptual and practical lessons derived from the scaling-up process will play a critical role in future efforts to expand and improve the quality of reproductive health services in Zambia.

Acknowledgements

The activities described in this chapter span nearly a decade and involve a cast of characters far too numerous to name, and far too important to describe in a sentence or two. Singling out individuals for special thanks is always fraught with peril, but it would be equally perilous to ignore the contributions of those who were truly indispensable in the successful transition from pilot to regional programme. These include the late Dr John Mbomena, team leader of the 1995 Zambia Contraceptive Needs Assessment and the inspiration for many of the activities described in this report; Dr Eddie Limbambala and Dr Simon

Miti, whose courage and, most importantly, willingness to exercise authority helped the pilot study overcome so many of the obstacles put before it; and Ms Tamara Fetters and Dr Miriam Chipimo, each of whom provided the technical guidance and programme oversight required to sustain the transition from the initial assessment to regional programme.

From assessment, to pilot study, to scaling up, USAID/Zambia and WHO were steadfast, sustaining the process, both financially and technically. They were joined in this effort by other key partners, such as the Population Council, CARE International, Georgetown University's Institute for Public Health, the Canadian Public Health Association, and of course the Zambia Ministry of Health, the Central Board of Health, the Copperbelt Provincial Health Office and the eight participating District Health Management Boards.

References

1. Fajans P, Simmons R, Ghiron L. Helping public sector health systems innovate: the strategic approach to strengthening reproductive health policies and programs. *American Journal of Public Health*, 2006, 96:435–440.

2. World Health Organization and Zambia Ministry of Health. *An assessment of the need for contraceptive introduction in Zambia. Research on the introduction and transfer of technologies for fertility regulation.* Geneva, UNDP/UNFPA/WHO/World Bank Special Programme of Research, Development and Research Training in Human Reproduction, 1995.

3. *Enhancing contraceptive choice and improving quality of family planning services in Zambia. Proceedings of dissemination workshop, Ndola, 25 January 2001.* Lusaka, Zambia Central Board of Health/Population Council/CARE International, 2001.

4. Muvandi I, Butrick E, Skibiak JP. *Measuring quality of care: a comparative analysis of situation analyses carried out in 1997 and 2000 under the Enhancing Contraceptive Choice and Improving Quality of Care Project.* Nairobi, The Population Council, 2001 (unpublished report).

5. Solo J, Luhanga M, Wohlfahrt D. Ready for change: a repositioning family planning case-study. New York, The ACQUIRE Project/EngenderHealth, 2005.

6. Korten DC, Klauss R, eds. *People-centered development: contributions toward theory and planning frameworks.* West Hartford, CT, Kumarian Press, 1984.

Chapter 5

Scaling up experimental project success with the Community-based Health Planning and Services initiative in Ghana

Frank K. Nyonator[a], Agyeman Badu Akosa[b], J. Koku Awoonor-Williams[c], James F. Phillips[d], Tanya C. Jones[e]

Summary

The Community-based Health Planning and Services (CHPS) initiative in Ghana is an example of a strategy for scaling up a field trial to become a national programme. Representing a response to the problem that research projects can inadvertently produce nonreplicable service delivery capabilities, CHPS develops mechanisms for expanding national understanding and use of research findings to serve the health service needs of all Ghanaian households. This chapter describes strategies for introducing and developing community health services that were successfully tested in a Navrongo Health Research Centre trial and validated in Nkwanta District for a national programme of reorienting primary health care from clinics to communities. Nurses, once confined to clinical duties, are relocated to community-constructed clinics where they live and work. Volunteers support their services by mobilizing traditional social institutions to foster community support. Strategies for decentralized planning ensure that operational details of the programme are adapted to local circumstances. Strengths and limitations of the programme are reviewed and discussed.

[a] Director, Policy Planning, Monitoring and Evaluation Division (PPMED), Ghana Health Service, Accra, Ghana. Dr Nyonator was formerly Regional Director of Medical Services, Volta Region, where he sponsored initial exchanges between Volta district teams and the Navrongo Health Research Centre that set the stage for the Community-based Health Planning and Services (CHPS) initiative.

[b] Director General, Ghana Health Service, Accra, Ghana. Dr Akosa directs the national programme of health sector reform, coordinating the process of converting CHPS innovations and policies into national action.

Footnotes continued on next page

Introduction

Clinic-focused services remain the mainstay of primary health care in Africa, despite several convincing demonstrations that community-based operations can enhance the accessibility, efficacy and sustainability of essential health services (1). While reforms are often proposed for changing national programmes from a clinic to a community-based focus, implementing such change requires a complex process for developing new structures, policies, resources and plans at each organizational level where change must be instituted. In the Republic of Ghana, policy commitment to achieving community-based care is not new (2). Deliberations on health sector reform began in the early 1980s but were given impetus in the 1990s by a continuous and growing role for research. The expanding influence of evidence-guided approaches was motivated by research showing that several large-scale national schemes focused on the need for accessible primary health care had been fraught with serious organizational problems and resource constraints (3). By 1990, achieving accessible primary health care had been a central pillar of policy for over a decade, yet the specific means of achieving this goal remained the subject of continuing discussion and debate.

This chapter reviews a national programme for reorienting and relocating primary health care from sub-district health centres to convenient community locations known as the Community-based Health Planning and Services (CHPS) initiative. The programme is grounded in evidence from a field trial of the Navrongo Health Research Centre showing that simple, low-cost services that engage the community can significantly reduce fertility and childhood mortality. The Navrongo Centre is well equipped to engage in health policy research. Located in Ghana's most impoverished and remote region, the Centre is a research unit of the Ministry of Health with a mandate to investigate

[c]   Director of Medical Services, Nkwanta District, Volta Region, Nkwanta, Ghana. Dr Awoonor-Williams directed the first replication of the Navrongo project in his home district and has led national exchanges among districts that spread programme innovations throughout Ghana, culminating in the creation of the Nkwanta Health Development Centre, where the principles of community health care are demonstrated to visiting health management teams.

[d]   Senior Associate, Policy Research Division, Population Council, New York, USA. Dr Phillips is Senior Adviser to the Navrongo project, and has extensive collaborative involvement with the CHPS monitoring and evaluation and communication activities.

[e]   Staff Associate, Policy Research Division of the Population Council, assigned as resident adviser to the PPMED, Ghana Health Service, Accra, Ghana. Ms Jones collaborates on organizational research and the administration of grants and awards to districts participating in the CHPS programme.

the health consequences of poverty and feasible means of addressing them. CHPS is a national initiative of the Ministry of Health that translates lessons from Navrongo research into national implementation of the long-standing Alma-Ata goal of "Health for All".

Phases in the scaling-up process

From the onset of planning, the Navrongo project was an instrument of the health sector reform process rather than a discrete research study for generating scientific results. The sustained partnership between researchers and policy-makers is portrayed in Figure 5.1 as a four-phased process guided by successive generations of research questions, approaches and products contributing to national health sector reform.

PHASE	POLICY DEBATE AND PILOT PROJECT 1990–1993	NAVRONGO TRIAL 1994–2000	NKWANTA VALIDATION 1998–2002	NATIONWIDE EXPANSION (CHPS) 2000–Present
QUESTION	What is appropriate?	Does it work?	Can it be validated?	Is scaling-up progressing?
APPROACH	Micro-pilot and social research	Factorial trial	Operations research	Quantitative and qualitative system appraisal
PRODUCT	Alternative models	Successful system	Consensus for change	Changed programme

Figure 5.1 Phases in the scaling-up process

Phase 1: policy debate and pilot

In Ghana, extending the coverage of basic and primary health-care services to all has been the major objective of the Ministry of Health since independence in 1957. Two general goals have guided primary health-care policy: the need to expand public sector health facilities, under the assumption that convenient facilities providing low-cost care will benefit the poor, and the need to shift resources from curative institution-based care to community-based preventive public health services. Although action in response to these goals produced notable results (4–6), impact of strategic change among the poorest segment of the population was disappointing (7).

Shortcomings in health service delivery were exacerbated by adverse worldwide economic shocks and the domestic economic problems of the 1980s. While external support increased owing to a proliferation of donor-led vertical health initiatives, the health sector was failing to meet the need for improved health-care coverage.

Launched in 1993, health sector reform in Ghana has aimed to increase access to services, improve health service quality and efficiency through decentralization of planning and management, foster partnerships between providers and communities, and expand health-care resources. Despite consensus on these goals, there has been long-standing debate on how to achieve them. Elements of this debate could not be resolved without a rigorous controlled trial of policy options. A 1991 order from the Director General of Medical Services created a task force to govern research and strategic decision-making. Chaired by the Director General, the task force was composed of the Director of Maternal and Child Health, the Director of the Health Research Unit, the Director of Public Health and the Director of the Navrongo Health Research Centre. A study protocol was drafted specifying scientific goals, activities, endpoints and mechanisms to ensure that evidence generated would guide large-scale reform. The approach was guided by international experience of linking innovators with policy-makers and sustaining evidence-based scaling up, even during periods of political and administrative change (8, Chapter 1).

Task force debate focused on the relative efficacy of two possible resources for implementing and governing accessible and affordable community health and family planning care. A view represented by the Bamako Initiative sponsored by the United Nations Children's Fund (UNICEF) emphasized the potential contribution of volunteer health providers and supporting cultural resources, such as chieftaincy, lineage and social network systems (9). In this perspective, vibrant traditional institutions for defining social structure, building consensus and establishing opinion leadership that are often ignored by health programmes could be utilized for developing sustainable volunteer health services. However, practical problems with implementing and managing volunteer programmes had been documented in the past (10, 11). In response to these problems, proponents of primary health care emphasized the potential impact of relocating underutilized community nurses to village locations (3). The task force prepared a protocol calling for a factorial trial to assess the relative childhood survival and fertility impact of marshalling two existing but underutilized resources for community health care. One arm of the study mobilized the health service capabilities of traditional leaders, social networks and volunteers; the other arm relocated underutilized community nurses from clinic locations to resident community health service delivery roles. Since strategies could be implemented independently, jointly, or not at all, the design implied four cells, with the comparison condition representing the existing clinic-focused system of care.

The trial was to be conducted by the Navrongo Health Research Centre in Kassena-Nankana District of the Upper East Region (see Figure 5.2) where high rates of malaria, respiratory disease, diarrhoeal disease, nutritional adversity and reproductive health morbidity produce high infant and child mortality. Fertility in the locality is high owing to gender stratification, low rates of literacy, extreme poverty and traditional beliefs that constrain the introduction of family planning services (12).

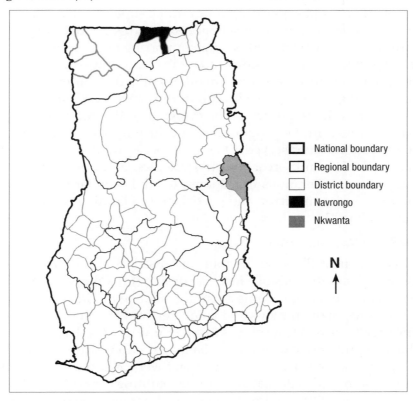

Figure 5.2 Map of the 10 regions and 110 districts of Ghana, highlighting the Kassena-Nankana District (Upper East Region) and Nkwanta District (Volta Region)

Phase 1 involved a pilot trial as well as social and operations research to clarify how the two experimental arms of the four-celled protocol could actually be implemented in such a challenging setting. In keeping with international experience in strategic planning, focus groups in three villages were convened to gauge opinion about the design of health and family planning services (13–16). Particular attention was directed to seeking guidance from women about their needs and advice on family planning service strategies. Activities emerged from these discussions that were implemented in a micro-pilot in three locations, focused on practical strategies for implementing the two experimental dimensions. Pilot activities were directed to developing guidelines for approaching chiefs and elders to engage their support and involvement in programme management, subordinating health leadership to the traditional system of community governance. Traditional leaders were oriented to the tasks of securing volunteer commitment to constructing community clinics, helping to solve the daily living needs of nurses, and supporting programme supervision and logistics operations. Pilot activities developed procedures for defining coverage areas of nurses, field methods for supporting nurse operations and training protocols for instructing nurses in community diplomacy. The pilot trial also focused on problems that applied to all experimental cells. For example, dialogue with community members aimed to identify ways to address gender problems, engage the support and participation of men in the programme, and sustain worker accountability to the communities served. Quarterly focus group sessions gauged worker and community reactions to strategies, permitting project scientists to revise operations in response to advice imparted (17). After 18 months of trial and error, and participatory planning, the task force launched Phase 2.

Phase 2: the Navrongo trial

To implement Phase 2, the four sub-districts of the district were randomized into the cells of a factorial design (18). Comparison of cells provided answers to questions about the relative merits of mobilizing traditional social institutions and volunteerism versus relocating community health nurses from clinics to communities. Results demonstrated that comprehensive community-based care was not only possible to achieve but also improved immunization coverage, service accessibility and the quantity of maternal and family planning care (19, 20). Putting a trained nurse in the community lessened parents' reliance on traditional healers when their children were sick (21) and reduced childhood mortality by more than a third (22). As the project progressed, community trust in nurses grew noticeably. Volunteers had no impact on parental health-seeking behaviour, however, because parents saw little distinction between the capabilities of traditional healers and volunteers (21). Nonetheless, volunteers played a crucial role in building the participation of men in family planning and developing gender outreach activities. In the final analysis, Navrongo was successful for all parameters examined, but child survival success was related solely to the performance of nurses, and family planning success was conditional on the joint work of community leaders, volunteers and nurses. Thus, the combined community nurse and volunteer cell was suggested and eventually adopted as the model for national policy.

Phase 3: the Nkwanta validation initiative

A National Dissemination Conference was convened in 1998 to disseminate preliminary Navrongo trial results. Participants included all senior health officials from national, regional and district levels. Debate ensued over the relevance of Navrongo to the national programme. Some participants argued that the unique institutional resources of the Navrongo Centre were responsible for project success and that these capabilities could not readily be replicated in rural settings that lacked resources for research. Others asserted that the process of observing workers, measuring results and interacting with communities had subtle and nonreplicable effects arising from the tendency of participants to view research activities as tantamount to supervisory oversight. Evidence of programme impact in Navrongo alone could not mobilize the political will essential for scaling up. Thus, there was a need to validate the Navrongo success story in other cultural and ecological zones of Ghana, using routinely available resources and mechanisms of the Ghana Health Service.

Early in 1998, the Volta Regional Health Administration initiated a field trip for orienting district directors to the Navrongo trial and expressed interest in testing the transfer of innovations to the relatively "normal" resource-constrained service setting of Nkwanta District. To build staff consensus, the Nkwanta District director of medical services, the public health nurse, two sub-district supervisors, and community nurses visited Navrongo to observe the project first hand. The team-building role of the field trip was crucial because Ghanaian social norms place a high value on collective decision-making. Fieldwork permitted open and frank discussion of nurses' concern that community posting would disrupt family life and social relations. In addition, supervisors had been clinic and office workers who seldom faced the rigours of community work. Since volunteers are not permitted to provide antibiotic therapy, some Volta Region medical officers expressed concern that involving volunteers in health services would divert health-seeking behaviour from comprehensive primary health care to the relatively ineffective clinical syndromic regimen that volunteers are allowed to provide. Anticipated administrative problems were also a source of apprehension. The logistics required to launch community services seemed daunting, particularly because community care would add to supervisory workloads rather than replace or restructure existing functions. The notion of mobilizing communities was perceived by some to be risky, since expectations might be aroused for non-sustainable levels of service intensity.

These matters were raised during direct exchange between individuals in the Navrongo team who had developed ways of solving them, and peer counterparts from Nkwanta seeking practical guidance. Field demonstration of service operations thus assured the Nkwanta team of the feasibility of restructuring health service delivery based on the Navrongo model. Nurses, in particular, welcomed interaction with Navrongo community nurses. The success of this exchange showed that transferring the Navrongo model to other districts is appropriately pursued by demonstration rather than by didactic classroom training. After a week of joint service delivery, Nkwanta staff members began to plan a two-community pilot that would adapt the Navrongo model to local circumstances and set the stage for intra-district peer exchanges where pilot teams would orient counterparts elsewhere in Nkwanta District. Nkwanta established the value of pilot adaptation of the Navrongo model, as opposed to mechanical replication of its operational details. The training programme subsequently developed by CHPS for district teams seeking to implement community-based care therefore focuses on methods for implementing pilot trials rather than procedures for implementing district-wide operations.

Results from the pilot demonstrated that the Navrongo model could be implemented with Nkwanta administrative systems and resources. Nkwanta is typical of the poorest localities in Ghana where contraceptive practice is rare and high childhood mortality results from high prevalence of measles, malaria and other communicable diseases and is compounded by the inaccessibility of health facilities and low rates of childhood immunization (23). A large isolated district spanning over 5500 km², Nkwanta has a subsistence economy based on agriculture and fishing. Ranking among the most impoverished districts in Ghana, Nkwanta lacks paved roads, communication infrastructure, and piped water. Educational attainment is low, particularly among women. Health services are rudimentary: a single physician serves 187 000 district residents and, when community health care was launched in 1999, there was no district hospital. Health staff typically were deployed to sub-district clinics located far from most communities, and outreach services were sporadic and poorly managed. Replicating the Navrongo model in such a setting, with the usual resources of a district management team, would represent a powerful endorsement of the relevance of the model to impoverished districts elsewhere in the country.

Though similar in development constraints and health problems, Navrongo and Nkwanta differ fundamentally in their cultural and ecological settings. Whereas Navrongo has two ethnolinguistic groups, each residing in dispersed settlement areas of geographically contiguous zones, Nkwanta settlement patterns are clustered by hamlet, each with multiple ethnolinguistic groups. As many as five languages may be spoken in a single village, with each group led by its own chieftaincy and lineage system. This linguistic diversity presents unique challenges for communication about behaviour change. Whereas Navrongo could rely upon councils of chiefs and elders for building community participation, the Nkwanta team relied upon respected non-traditional leaders and groups, such as teachers, elected officials and faith-based organizations, to build consensus for the programme among traditional leaders. Finally, while Navrongo has extensive resources for equipment and logistics support embedded in its research protocol, Nkwanta's less sophisticated institutional capacity is more typical of district health systems in other rural districts of Ghana. The Nkwanta team developed management information procedures for tracking births and immunizations that could be implemented without computer technology.

The validation exercise in Nkwanta demonstrated that implementing community-based services would require substantial changes in the health-care system and identified the operational details of phasing in community health services community by community over time. Steps developed in Navrongo for changing operations from clinic-focused to community-based services were clarified, documented and validated by the Nkwanta District Health Management Team, resulting in the following six major sequential milestones (Table 5.1):

1. **Preliminary planning**, which involves grouping communities into service zones, specifying where each nurse is assigned to provide care, identifying community leaders and planning optimal location of the facilities to be used as service points for community-based health care (health compounds);

2. **Community entry**, which includes conducting meetings and diplomacy with village leaders, convening public gatherings, known as durbars, for communicating plans and activities to communities, and constituting health liaison committees for providing daily support to the programme;

3. **Health compound construction**, which utilizes volunteer labour and community resources to develop the dwelling unit where nurses live and work;

4. **Procurement of essential equipment**, such as motorbikes, bicycles and clinical equipment;

5. **Posting nurses,** and providing them with technical refresher training and orientation to communities where they are assigned;

6. **Volunteer recruitment**, which involves engaging health committees in designating health volunteers to assist with community activities in child health, family planning and other reproductive health services.

| Milestone | Type of operation | | Implementation tasks |
	Existing clinic-based system	Community-based services	
Planning	District Health Management Team; office-based planning	Defined community service areas, termed zones; traditional leaders; community nurses	Community mapping and enumeration; outreach to traditional leaders
Community entry	None	Community leadership support for health services; community health committees for governing operations	Community awareness building, liaison with leaders; community health committee selection; training of community nurse for community entry; community leadership training
Community health compound	None (sub-district health centre and hospital services)	Community constructed or refurbished nurse service and dwelling units; community ownership of primary service point	Community mobilization for facility development; community support for maintenance
Essential equipment	Four-wheel vehicle for biweekly outreach clinics (rarely available); sub-district and district hospital equipment	Bicycles or motorbikes for continuous outreach by nurse; basic clinical equipment for community health compounds	Procurement of bicycles, motorbikes, and basic community clinical equipment

Milestone	Type of operation		Implementation tasks
	Existing clinic-based system	Community-based services	
Nurse posting	Nurses resident at the sub-district or district level; sub-district health centre-based services; passive (facility-focused); biweekly/ monthly outreach clinics at fixed locations	Community resident nurses providing static services based in community health compound augmented by active (client-seeking) outreach to families in their homes	Supervisory provision of fuel for household visitation activities and supplies for clinical work; supervisory community backstopping of nursing operations; community support for operations; in-service training for nurses; motorbike rider training and maintenance capacity building
Volunteer deployment	None	Selection by traditional leaders and community health committees; supervision by community health committees; training by district health management team	Train community leaders in volunteer recruitment and management; train community health committees to select and supervise volunteers; train volunteers

Table 5.1 Milestones in establishing community-based services by type of operational change required in the scaling-up process

At least 20 specific component activities have also been identified, though their sequence of implementation differs from locality to locality.

The process of transfer also demonstrated ways in which the strategy for expansion could improve upon the Navrongo model. Changes in the Navrongo approach to community mobilization were introduced to respond to ethnic diversity, which is common in southern Ghana but rare in the northern regions. Moreover, volunteers were deployed as community health organizers rather than as front-line service providers, in response to Navrongo research showing that child health is not improved by volunteer service delivery (21, 22).

Surveys conducted in 1999 and 2002 suggest that the validation effort had succeeded. In the 1999 baseline survey, family planning usage in Nkwanta District was estimated to be less than 4% (23). By 2002, prevalence was 14% in communities exposed to the programme, representing three times the prevailing rates in the rest of the district. Similarly, the odds of knowing at least one method of family planning were 2.2 times greater than among other district residents. Health indicators were also affected. The odds of having received antenatal care were more than five times greater among women residing in service communities than for others. Postnatal care odds were four times greater, and the odds of receiving both antenatal and postnatal care were greater as well.

Nkwanta not only validated Navrongo effects, but exceeded Navrongo levels of impact on several health indicators (23). Some elements of the Nkwanta service delivery system, however, did not achieve the same degree of success. Service components that benefit from sophisticated technical operations like those found in Navrongo are not easily replicated with routine service statistics. For example, childhood immunization services benefit from accurate and timely data on pregnancy and delivery, since the timing of immunization in infancy is crucial to the efficacy of each modality. Non-computerized procedures in Nkwanta have yet to achieve fully the precision and efficiency of the Navrongo system. While active outreach should result in higher immunization coverage than passive fixed posts or mobile clinic approaches, the Nkwanta experience demonstrated that vaccination coverage was not enhanced for all antigens, suggesting that impact is contingent on improved management information systems that support the prioritization of activities and correct timing of immunization for each infant served. In response to these findings, Nkwanta has developed a new information system for immunization that will be more appropriate for other districts than the Navrongo system.

Nkwanta was crucial for initiating the national scaling-up process by demonstrating that: 1) transfer of the service model from a research project to a district health service operation is possible, even in a challenging setting; 2) adapting and refining the underlying service model in a demonstration district is both necessary and feasible if low-cost research tools are used to generate evidence; and 3) scaling up involves a transfer of the service model to new districts through peer training for pilot teams followed by subsequent pilots and peer exchanges within implementing districts. In response to this success, the Ghana Health Service utilizes Nkwanta as a demonstration district for building CHPS implementation capacity.

Phase 4: nationwide expansion

A 1999 National Health Forum focused on the Nkwanta experience. Practical guidelines for implementing community services were presented and discussed, and consensus emerged that national implementation of the Navrongo service model was feasible. A consensus document, approved by acclamation at the Forum, led to the launching of the Community-based Health Planning and Services initiative in 2000, a programme for scaling up based on lessons from the Navrongo and Nkwanta experience. Three overarching features of CHPS govern its strategic design: policy, evidence and action.

Policy. Meetings, staff conferences, field exchanges, policies, plans and directives from headquarters catalyse and legitimize nationwide expansion at all levels of the Ghana Health Service. CHPS-sponsored field exchanges have been designed to build consensus and commitment for action. Newsletters from Navrongo and Nkwanta communicate to all district teams practical lessons and experience so that district plans benefit from advice from the field. National policies, in turn, legitimize the process of operational change, producing budgets and manpower assessments that respond to the requirements of a highly decentralized programme of action. Manpower shortages represent the key challenge to national health plans, and expansion of the community nurse workforce is now a major Ghana Health Service priority. Strategies are in the offing for new training schools, new approaches to training and in-service training activities. Ghana Health Service commitment to the initiative ensures that resources will be marshalled to support manpower expansion, and that the overall quality of healthcare delivery will be improved as community services are scaled up as a national programme.

Evidence. The programme marshals evidence to evaluate whether strategies developed in Navrongo and Nkwanta can be scaled up with replicable levels of success. Regional and national staff meetings and Annual National Health Forum Conferences provide mechanisms for discussion of monitoring and evaluation results among health managers at all levels in the Ghana Health Service. In this manner "bottom-up" and "top-down" communication systems integrate evidence into routine management decision-making. The generation of the following three types of evidence ensures that no one type of data, source of learning or research paradigm dominates.

First, a programme of qualitative research, involving focus-groups with community leaders and members, front-line workers, supervisors, district managers, local politicians and administrators, elicits perceptions of progress and problems at each level of service delivery. Sessions are conducted by Regional Health Administration study teams, with technical support from the Policy Planning, Monitoring and Evaluation Division (PPMED) of the Ghana Health Service. This approach sacrifices an element of objectivity but sets the stage for dissemination of results at senior Ghana Health Service managers' meetings.

Second, district CHPS implementation checklists record the coverage, content and pace of programme expansion in quarterly reports from each of the 110 districts in Ghana. Data are managed by PPMED, and quarterly reports to all district, regional and national health officials provide maps of progress, data on the status of implementation, newsletters and all existing diagnostic research reports.[1] The monitoring system generates national planning data as well as information for stakeholders about progress on all implementation indicators.

Third, survey data record impact statistics in districts where CHPS implementation is advanced. Geographical variation in community health service coverage permits PPMED to conduct surveys that demonstrate the potential contribution of CHPS to health development in Ghana (for example, 24, 25). These studies, which are dispersed throughout all regions of Ghana, have determined that Nkwanta results are evident in every setting where CHPS has been implemented (26).

Action. Each region has established a demonstration district where the approach is put to a test and adapted as needed. "Guided diffusion" stimulates operational change offsetting some of the resource requirements of scaling up. (27–29). The exchange process of transferring Navrongo learning to Nkwanta pilot teams and subsequent community exchanges within Nkwanta District provided a model of peer training that guides national expansion.

Peer training involves posting district teams to counterparts for two weeks of collaborative fieldwork, problem solving and planning. Nurses working with nurses, and supervisors working with counterparts, are introduced to all practical steps so they are aware of the elements of operational change inherent in implementing the six milestones (see Table 5.1). Typically, trainee teams are composed of the implementation hierarchy required for starting a two-zone pilot: the District Director of Health Services, the Public Health Nurse, the District CHPS Coordinator, one or two sub-district supervisors and the Community Health Officer (nurse) from the pilot sub-district. In this approach, structured interaction between district teams breaks down isolation, confusion and ambivalence about the initiative, while interaction among community leaders within implementing districts facilitates learning once the change process has been launched.

---

[1] See http://www.ghana-chps.org

Sites for Nkwanta-like orientations are being expanded through competitive grants sponsored by the Population Council to district teams that have demonstrated advanced CHPS implementation capabilities. Small grants fund the evaluation of innovations to the programme and the cost of orienting visiting district teams in implementing innovation elsewhere. Thirteen districts have received awards, each providing funds for training teams from six other districts.

Peer training has been augmented with technical training for developing service quality, referral services and supervisory support. A Ghana Health Service technical training team conducts quality assurance field appraisals and in-service training as needed. New manuals, protocols and procedures have been developed for ensuring technical standards in community health nursing.

Peer training commences once technical training has been completed. Pilot work zones are used for orienting neighbouring community leaders to the programme. Durbars are used to build public awareness about the benefits of the programme. Awareness typically spreads to neighbouring communities, and political commitment to the initiative grows. This sometimes leads to District Assembly commitment of development revenue for community health compound costs (24).

In national policy documents, CHPS is viewed as a mechanism for integrating activities of the formal health sector into traditional institutions that define community leadership, foster consensus building and sustain collective action. Research reports provided highly credible evidence supporting policy commitment to this model. Such evidence has been a determinant of successful scaling up elsewhere (Chapter 1).

Constraints to scaling up

The CHPS initiative has made considerable progress. Only 22 of 110 districts reported implementing activities at the beginning of 2001; 18 months later, 87 districts had taken steps to launch the programme. By mid-2004, 105 of the 110 District Health Management Teams reported having undertaken preliminary planning activities. Although nearly every district in Ghana has joined the scaling-up process, a number of obstacles have emerged. The pace of launching programme planning has progressed more rapidly than the pace of implementing community-based services. Although approximately two thirds of the districts report having completed community-based planning, relatively few have actually launched services. At the beginning of 2003, only 42% of the districts had completed the process of community entry in at least one service zone, even though community entry is a low-cost and simple-to-implement strategic component of the programme. A greater proportion of zones had completed Community Health Compound construction or renovation, suggesting that facilities are being developed without community involvement, and that community posting of the nurse or volunteer development lags behind all other milestones. This commitment of district resources for construction, without resource leveraging from communities, represents a departure from the CHPS model of community engagement that deprives the programme of community resources for facilities and community ownership of the programme itself. Qualitative systems appraisals show that communities which mobilize resources for the programme develop a sense of ownership of its services. Constructing facilities without community engagement is tantamount to bypassing social support for CHPS in general.

Staff engaged in the programme tend to be supportive of CHPS, but workers who are not familiar with the initiative resist its introduction (30). The following three themes explain this reluctance:

The knowledge gap. CHPS continues to mean different things to different stakeholders, despite the considerable effort that has been directed to training, policy directives, conferences and reports. In its simplest distortion, the programme is viewed as a means of putting nurses into communities, and little else. Because health workers at all levels are accustomed to clinic-based work routines, instructions to relocate nurses to communities get interpreted through the prism of clinic management experience. Front-line workers often amplify managerial concerns about the feasibility of shifting operations from clinics to communities. Nurses who are relocated to communities must leave behind the relative comfort of sub-district assignments, where work is routinely supervised and technical demands are minimal. Nurses express concern about the challenge ahead and managers are anxious about embarking upon changes that may be complicated to manage. Many of the key staff involved in decision-making have responsibility for clinical roles and little extra time for organizing community health care. While the potential difficulties of launching CHPS are anticipated, compensating benefits are not readily understood. By contrast, workers actually participating in the programme express satisfaction about their contribution to health service improvements and their appreciation of the support that communities render (31).

The resource gap. Resources for primary health care in Ghana are severely constrained. Increasing the coverage of community health services expands demand for health care that translates into higher costs of pharmaceuticals, fuel, equipment and supplies. Health sector reform has conferred authority on district health management teams, but has not provided the necessary resources for implementing the general health service agenda. In the absence of earmarked donor or government funding for CHPS, incremental start-up costs severely constrain efforts to launch the programme. Given the financial and manpower limitations confronting districts, many are understandably reluctant to engage in "community entry" activities that will arouse public interest in services they are ill-equipped to launch and sustain.

The technical gap. District health management teams are often reluctant to launch a programme that they believe will require technical skills not yet in place. Management information systems, logistics systems and community outreach operations lack essential tools for ensuring that quality services will be maintained and that community health-care delivery will adequately respond to community needs. Community nurses often are ill equipped to make independent clinical decisions, having grown accustomed to the continuous technical supervision that sub-district health centres afford. Once they are deployed to communities they immediately confront major technical challenges. For example, communities typically expect arriving nurses to have midwifery skills that few are trained and equipped to provide. CHPS requires new training protocols and procedures that are not yet in place.

Responding to constraints

What is being done to solve these problems? Contrasting the responses of leading districts with those slow to implement operational change suggests the following possible solutions:

Responding to the knowledge gap. As the Nkwanta experience demonstrated, peer exchange resolves conceptual confusion by exposing participants to the practical requirements of changing operations. This type of training, originally provided in Nkwanta and Navrongo, is being extended to other advanced CHPS districts. A more extensive field demonstration programme is under development that will provide each of the regions with at least one Nkwanta-like demonstration district. In the past, technical training has been provided through workshops for individual nurses that were unconnected with field demonstration activities for district implementation teams. The CHPS demonstration programme will be augmented with a new in-service technical training component for upgrading clinical skills that are needed for service provision, referral, quality assurance and community-based health management. The integration of nurse training with team demonstration will ensure that scaling up improves rather than dilutes service quality.

Responding to resource constraints. CHPS implementation follows the principles of the diffusion of innovation. Districts are administrative units that foster interaction of workers within district boundaries, but also constrain interaction among workers of different districts. Therefore, scaling up spreads within districts once the initiative gets started in one or two zones, but spreads slowly across district boundaries *(32)*. Catalysing the diffusion process requires investment in trials in pilot zones that demonstrate CHPS within districts and set the stage for community-to-community diffusion of innovation. Experimentation with these mechanisms remains nascent, but they involve constituting all milestones of the CHPS programme in pilot areas and inviting leaders from neighbouring communities to participate in durbars, observe service operations and witness community commitment. The Nkwanta experience showed that such exchanges fostered the spread of health action and volunteerism, offsetting the costs of developing and sustaining the programme.

Moreover, districts progressing with scaling up have developed creative ways of solving resource constraints. Two districts have marshalled district assembly support and development funds for augmenting programme revenue. Others have raised donations through community activities and faith-based organizations. One district has developed creative ways to solve manpower problems with "private practitioners" – paramedics who are financed by the community rather than salaried employees of the Ghana Health Service. Field investigation consistently shows that rapidly advancing districts have developed innovative strategies for solving resource constraints.

There is reason to doubt that community commitment alone can fill the resource gap, however. The "Common Fund" of health sector reform commits only US$ 6.80 per capita per year to district revenue, and this commitment covers the full range of preventive and ambulatory services. If CHPS is to progress, added revenue will be required, at least for financing pilots that start operations. In Navrongo, US$ 1.92 per capita per year is required, over and above routine district revenue. Nkwanta has cost less, but even in that district, scaling up would not have started without the catalytic contribution of two Navrongo motorbikes and US$ 12 000-worth of supplies and equipment from a faith-based charity. At the very least, a commitment of this magnitude will be required to launch and sustain pilot activities that enable district teams to get CHPS started without delay, mobilize community support for the programme by demonstrating its potential, and build staff understanding of how to make the programme work. Just as CHPS demonstrates that communities will finance a community-based programme, its slow pace of expansion demonstrates that well-placed development investment is essential to accelerating the scaling-up process.

Responding to manpower and technical gaps. Evidence suggesting that nurses often fear community deployment has raised fundamental questions about manpower policy. Community Health Nurses are trained in one of four national training schools, fees are paid by the government, and graduates are deployed to sub-districts by central order. Much of the concern that nurses express about community deployment derives from the obvious fact that they are not from communities where they will live and work, may not speak the local language, and may be compelled to live separately from families and kin. To deal with these problems, Navrongo has launched a "community engaged" approach to decentralized training. Communities select nurse trainees, who are sent to a local training centre where fees are paid by the districts and communities to be served by the trainees. Upon graduation, nurses return home, rather than to a post in a distant location. Evidence from this trial has generated new policies for the national nurse training programme. Ten new decentralized schools are being opened; 10 more are planned with the goal of scaling up the availability of trained manpower and improving the quality and social relevance of CHPS manpower policies. This experience attests to the importance of continuous investigation and revision of scaling-up policy as initiatives mature.

Conclusion

Despite the challenges that have been identified, the CHPS initiative has begun to introduce health-care reform in every region of Ghana. Much remains to be accomplished, but concepts guiding the initiative have been tested in Navrongo and shown to be fundamentally sound. Various principles of scaling up have been demonstrated by this experience. In Ghana, scaling up has been a process of organizational change and development that required working in phases guided by evidence. The role and type of research shifted as the programme progressed, not only guiding the continuous process of expansion and development, but also identifying problems and permitting strategic change and improvement as scaling up progressed.

Scaling up in Ghana has derived particular benefit from replication and validation studies. Nkwanta validated the notion that the Navrongo approach could work elsewhere, and demonstrated that the Navrongo model is less a prescription for replication than a generic process for adaptive development of appropriate health care that could work in other areas of Ghana. Further replication initiatives have confirmed and legitimized the rationale for programme expansion. Scaling up the programme beyond Nkwanta required specific guidelines on components of the clinical programme that required change, steps required in the process of operational change, and procedures for monitoring whether organizational change was actually taking place. While replication projects have strengthened commitment to CHPS, sustaining Navrongo has provided a continuing resource for demonstrating the model, promoting its worth and documenting the evidence on which the national scaling-up initiative is based. If the Ghana Health Service had abandoned Navrongo when CHPS was launched, scaling up would have lost the wisdom, commitment and capabilities of its founding implementation team. The Ghana example demonstrates not only the value of replication projects, but also the continuing value of the founding project in dissemination, training and advocacy.

Large-scale programme expansion in Ghana has been guided by multiple sources of evidence and sustained by complementary strategies for communicating results to stakeholders. Monitoring activities record both qualitative information on programme problems and quantitative data on the spread of programme activities. Evidence gathered through a range of activities and experience with the initiative has fostered decentralized planning, training and adaptive development of strategies to local circumstances and needs. The accumulation of evidence has been combined with communication activities for ensuring that results are put to use. Newsletters document community and worker experience with the programme. Conferences, demonstration exchanges and staff meetings build consensus and understanding of the initiative and sustain the scaling-up process.

CHPS is thus a complex story. Its core strategy is based on an elaborate experiment, multiple replication efforts and diverse sources of evidence. Its core agenda, however, is quite simple for stakeholders to understand and embrace. If CHPS succeeds, it will have demonstrated mechanisms for bringing health services to every Ghanaian doorstep by aligning health sector policy, evidence and action with vibrant social traditions of community leadership, communication and volunteerism.

Acknowledgements

The authors gratefully acknowledge the many dedicated Ghana Health Service workers who have made, and continue to make, CHPS a success. In particular, we thank the scientists and service workers of the Navrongo Health Research Centre and Nkwanta District Health Administration who set the stage for the CHPS initiative. This work was made possible through grants to the Population Council and sub-awards to the Ghana Health Service funded by the United States Agency for International Development. Rockefeller Foundation grants to the Navrongo Health Research Centre funded demographic research and Ghana Health Service dissemination conferences that led to the CHPS initiative.

References

1. *Better health in Africa: experiences and lessons learned.* Washington, DC, The World Bank, 1994.

2. *The Danfa comprehensive rural health and family planning project: summary, conclusions, and recommendations from the final report.* Accra, University of Ghana Medical School, 1979 (unpublished).

3. Amonoo-Larsen R, Ebrahim G, Lovel H et al. *District health care: challenges for planning, organization and evaluation in developing countries.* London, Macmillan Press, 1984.

4. *Medium-term health strategy* (September 1995). Accra, Ministry of Health of the Republic of Ghana, 1995.

5. *The health of the nation: reflections on the first five-year health sector programme of work, 1997–2001.* Accra, Ministry of Health of the Republic of Ghana, 2001.

6. *Fourth review under the poverty reduction and growth facility, requests for waiver of performance criteria and for extension of the commitment period.* Accra, International Monetary Fund, 2002 (unpublished report by the African Department).

7. *A profile of health inequities in Ghana.* Accra, Ministry of Health of the Republic of Ghana, 1998.

8. Akosa BA, Nyonator FK, Phillips JF et al. *Health sector reform, field experiments, and systems research for evidence-based programme change and development in Ghana.* Paper prepared for: From Pilot Projects to Policies and Programmes, Rockefeller Foundation Conference, Bellagio Study and Conference Center, 31 March–5 April 2003.

9. Knippenberg R, Levy-Bruhl D, Osseni R et al. *The Bamako Initiative: primary health care.* New York, United Nations Children's Fund, 1990.

10. Agyepong IA, Marfo C. Internal evaluation of the Dangme West District Village Health Worker Programme. Accra, Ministry of Health of the Republic of Ghana, 1992 (unpublished, Health Research Unit).

11.   Agyepong IA. Reforming health service delivery at district level in Ghana: the perspective of a district medical officer. *Health Policy and Planning*, 1999, 14:59–69.

12.   Adongo PB, Phillips JF, Kajihara BZ et al. Cultural factors constraining the introduction of family planning among the Kassena-Nankana of northern Ghana. *Social Science and Medicine*, 1997, 45:1789–1804.

13.   Korten D. Community organization and rural development: a learning process approach. *Public Administration Review*, 1980, 40:480–511.

14.   Simmons R, Phillips JF, Rahman M. Strengthening government health and family planning programmes: findings from an action research project in Bangladesh. *Studies in Family Planning*, 1984, 15:212–221.

15.   Simmons R, Hall P, Díaz J et al. The strategic approach to contraceptive introduction. *Studies in Family Planning*, 1997, 28:79–94.

16.   Simmons R, Brown J, Díaz M. Facilitating large-scale transitions to quality of care: an idea whose time has come. *Studies in Family Planning*, 2002, 33:61–75.

17.   Nazzar A, Adongo PB, Binka F et al. Involving a traditional community in strategic planning: the Navrongo community health and family planning project pilot study. *Studies in Family Planning*, 1995, 26:307–324.

18.   Binka FN, Nazzar A, Phillips JF. The Navrongo community health and family planning project. *Studies in Family Planning*, 1995, 26:121–139.

19.   Debpuur C, Phillips JF, Jackson EF et al. The impact of the Navrongo project on contraceptive knowledge and use, reproductive preferences, and fertility. *Studies in Family Planning*, 2002, 33:141–164.

20.   Phillips JF, Jackson EF, Bawah AA et al. *The fertility impact of the Navrongo project*. Paper presented at: Population Association of America Annual Meeting, Minneapolis, MN, April 2003.

21.   Nyarko P, Pence B, Adongo P. *Child morbidity and health-seeking behaviour of primary caretakers in the Kassena-Nankana District of northern Ghana*. Accra, Ministry of Health of the Republic of Ghana, 2004 (unpublished).

22.   Nyarko P, Pence B, Phillips JF et al. *The impact of the Navrongo community health and family planning project on child mortality, 1995–2000*. New York, The Population Council, 2005 (Policy Research Division Working Paper).

23. Awoonor-Williams JK, Feinglass ES, Tobey R et al. The impact of a replication project on safe motherhood and family planning behavior in Nkwanta District of Ghana. *Studies in Family Planning*, 2004, 35:161–177.

24. Antwi P, Nyonator FK, Jones TC et al. *The impact of the community-based health planning and services (CHPS) program on maternal health in the Abura-Asebu Kwamankese District in Ghana.* Paper presented at: Population Association of America Annual Meeting, Boston, MA, 1–3 April 2004.

25. Kuffour E, Antwi P, Nyonator FK. *Programme evaluation when there is purposive placement: an example of a social programme in Ghana.* Accra, Ghana Health Service, 2004 (Policy Planning, Monitoring and Evaluation Division, unpublished).

26. Nyonator FK, Phillips JF, Vaughan-Smith M. *The health and family planning impact of the community-based health planning and services initiative in nine rural districts of Ghana.* Accra, Ghana Health Service, 2005 (Report of the Policy Planning, Monitoring and Evaluation Division).

27. Glaser EM, Abelson HH, Garrison KN. *Putting knowledge to use: facilitating the diffusion of knowledge and the implementation of planned change.* San Francisco, CA, Jossey-Bass Inc., 1983.

28. Rogers EM. *Diffusion of innovations*, 4th ed. New York, Free Press, 1995.

29. Mintrom M. Policy entrepreneurs and the diffusion of innovation. *American Journal of Political Science*, 1997, 41:738–770.

30. Nyonator FK, Jones TC, Miller RA et al. Guiding the Ghana Community-based Health Planning and Services approach to scaling up with qualitative systems appraisal. *International Quarterly of Community Health Education*, 2005, 23:189–213.

31. Sory EK, Jones TC, Nyonator FK et al. *Grassroots mobilization to accelerate the introduction of community-based health service delivery in Ghana: strategic assessment of the CHPS program in the central region of Ghana.* Paper presented at: American Public Health Association Annual Meeting, San Francisco, CA, 15–19 November 2003.

32. Nyonator FK, Awoonor-Williams JK, Phillips JF et al. The Ghana Community-based Health Planning and Services initiative: fostering evidence-based organizational change and development in a resource-constrained setting. *Health Policy and Planning*, 2005, 20:25–34.

Chapter 6

Evidence-based scaling up of health and family planning service innovations in Bangladesh and Ghana

James F. Phillips[a], Frank K. Nyonator[b], Tanya C. Jones[c], Shruti Ravikumar[d]

Summary

This chapter describes two initiatives that have utilized research to guide the development and scaling up of community-based health and family planning programmes. In Bangladesh and Ghana, evidence was accumulated in stages, beginning with an exploratory investigation, followed by an experimental trial testing potential interventions and a replication phase for validating research results in a non-research programme setting. The process concluded with research-guided programme expansion. Each stage was associated with shifts in generations of questions, mechanisms and outcomes as the process unfolded. Large-scale health systems development was achieved in both countries, not because the scaling-up strategies were alike but because similar research approaches led to different strategies adapted to contrasting societal and institutional contexts.

[a] Senior Associate, Policy Research Division, the Population Council, New York, USA. Dr Phillips is Senior Adviser to the Navrongo Experiment, and has extensive collaborative involvement with the Community-based Health Planning and Services (CHPS) monitoring and evaluation and communication activities.

[b] Director, Policy Planning, Monitoring and Evaluation Division (PPMED), Ghana Health Service, Accra, Ghana. Dr Nyonator was formerly Regional Director of Medical Services, Volta Region, where he sponsored initial exchanges between Volta district teams and the Navrongo Health Research Centre that set the stage for the CHPS initiative.

[c] Staff Associate, Policy Research Division, the Population Council, assigned as resident adviser to the PPMED, Ghana Health Service, Accra, Ghana. Ms Jones collaborates on organizational research and the administration of grants and awards to districts participating in the CHPS programme.

[d] Shruti Ravikumar is a student at the Yale Law School and an intern at the Population Council. She conducted the literature review for this study.

Introduction

Over the last three decades, successive international initiatives have focused on the problem of making reproductive and child health services accessible to the poor: Alma-Ata's "Health for All" in the 1980s, the Integrated Management of Childhood Illness in the 1990s, the 1994 International Conference for Population and Development, in Cairo, and more recently the Millennium Development Goals. National implementation of these initiatives has typically been pursued through central policy directives rather than based on evidence from the communities to be served. As a consequence, low-cost effective technologies that could substantially reduce reproductive and child health morbidity and mortality remain inaccessible to the rural poor (1, 2). Promising health service models are sometimes demonstrated by research, but the relevance of research-based success to large-scale action is often brought into question by researchers' access to special resources and flexibility to manage and lead small-scale projects.

This chapter compares two community health and family planning case-studies where major health system changes used research as a tool for developing national reform as bottom-up rather than top-down initiatives: the Matlab and Extension projects in Bangladesh and the Navrongo and Community-based Health Planning and Services (CHPS) projects in Ghana. These initiatives introduced important systems changes that were tested at the community level, found to work and then scaled up in an evidence-guided process of national reform.

The application of a similar process in contrasting settings

The Bangladesh and Ghana cases addressed the challenging question of how to deliver maternal health and family planning services in settings where service provision and utilization were constrained by social, geographical and economic factors. Both instituted a multi-year process using a similar evidence-based approach for resolving debate about policy options, and for guiding programme development and scaling up. Research was crucial to this process, with four successive phases designed to focus on policy and programme development. First, preliminary qualitative appraisal was used to diagnose problems and develop strategies for experimental trial. Second, experimental trials were organized to test the demographic impact of strategic change. Successful trials generated questions about the broader relevance of results leading to the third phase of investigation that tested transferability of experimental operations to the national programme. Evidence from this third phase was used to build consensus for national reform and strategies for implementing scaling-up activities. The fourth and final phase utilized research for monitoring the progress of scaling up, the coverage of changed operations, and problems hampering change and reform. In these settings, the generation and utilization of evidence was an integral component of programme development rather than an end in itself. The consistent focus on evidence enabled policy-makers and programme managers to develop service strategies that were appropriate for the social and institutional context. Since contexts varied, this similar process generated very different programmes and scaling-up approaches in the two countries.

The Bangladesh case

In the early 1970s, at the time of Bangladesh's independence, prospects that health services could reduce fertility or mortality were the subject of international debate. The clinical efficacy of various technologies, such as childhood immunization, was well known. Pervasive economic, health and nutritional adversity at the time of independence, however, led to synergistic disease risks that could offset the benefits of specific technologies (3, 4). High fertility was the consequence of pronatalist social institutions (5, 6). There was no evidence that family planning services would reduce fertility in this context. Yet the newly constituted Government of Bangladesh assigned priority to developing a national family planning programme, a policy that was met with considerable international scepticism and debate (7).

In 1975, the International Centre for Diarrhoeal Disease Research, Bangladesh (ICDDR,B), now known as the Centre for Health and Population Research, launched investigations designed to guide national population policy. ICDDR,B's Matlab field station was chosen for these investigations because it was located in a traditional, rural and isolated locality where the demographic transition had not begun, and where challenges confronting effective family planning service delivery were typical of vast areas of deltaic Bangladesh. Matlab's comprehensive demographic research system had been used to study a wide range of social, demographic and epidemiological issues (8). Owing to the availability of these unique research resources in a challenging social, health and economic context, the site was ideal for resolving policy debate on whether family planning services could work in this society.

Initial experimental research, launched in 1975 as the Contraceptive Distribution Project, focused on testing the demographic impact of distributing oral contraceptive supplies through doorstep outreach to married women. No attempt was made to assess social perceptions of family planning, the acceptability of oral contraception, or health needs more generally. There was also no attempt to provide other contraceptive options, counselling or quality safeguards. When the project failed to have impact (9), Matlab managers, supervisors and researchers launched a series of qualitative studies to diagnose the reasons for failure. This investigation noted strong adverse community reactions to the project's focus on oral contraceptives and its lack of maternal and child health services. It also identified poor worker training and poor interactions with clients and communities more generally. Discussion of results provided a crucial source of social learning about community preferences and needs (10).

In the subsequent Family Planning and Health Services Project, evidence generated by the appraisal was used to develop strategies for correcting deficiencies of the failed initial project. Uneducated traditional birth attendants were replaced by educated, young married women who were locally recruited. These field workers visited married women every two weeks to consult with them about their family planning needs and their health. They were provided with on-the-job training in basic health and family planning care and referral services, and had medical backup and support from supervisors when problems arose. Contraceptive choice was expanded so that couples selecting a contraceptive method had multiple options. Child health and basic primary health services were developed, ensuring that outreach and referral covered the most extensive range of services the programme could provide, including treatment for febrile illnesses, management of diarrhoeal diseases and referral to paramedical care at nearby health centres. This broadened provision of care led researchers to extend the scope of enquiry to include questions about the impact of community health services on child survival.

Providing women with expanded contraceptive choices and quality services increased their satisfaction and contraceptive prevalence. By 1980, the early fertility impact of the Matlab Project was pronounced (11) and the health service components of the project improved child survival (12). These findings – disseminated in meetings and professional papers – suggested that national health goals could be achieved with community-based approaches if staffing, training and deployment schemes in the national programme were modelled on the Matlab Project.

Despite its demographic success, and widespread discussion of the results, the Matlab Project had no immediate policy impact. During a 1981 tripartite review sponsored by the United Nations, the Bangladesh Government rejected the proposition that Matlab results could be taken at face value as a model for the national programme. They argued that the experiment had more service delivery staff, more financial resources and a different service regimen than the national programme. Replicating its operational design on a large scale would require major organizational change. Following this review, policy debate shifted from the question about whether the Matlab service system could succeed to the question of whether successful strategies were replicable within the national programme.

To resolve policy debate, senior government officials proposed a validation study that would test the transferability of Matlab's comprehensive integrated health and family planning approach to localities where service delivery was conducted with usual government health sector staff, mechanisms and resources. Such a study, known as the Maternal and Child Health and Family Planning Extension Project, was organized by the ICDDR,B in districts located in regions distant from the Matlab field station. In two districts, Matlab scientists, supervisors and other ICDDR,B staff served as a resource team that provided training and technical support to the government staff (13, 14). Matlab primary health-care staff and supervisors were assigned to the intervention areas to work for three months as counterparts to government workers. Two neighbouring districts served as comparison areas.

Research results soon demonstrated that there were major obstacles to implementing the Matlab approach within the government programme. For example, longitudinal survey data showed that Matlab effects were replicated when client–worker exchanges occurred. The frequency of these encounters in Extension Project areas was low, however, because the catchment population for a given worker was six times larger than that of a fieldworker in Matlab (15). Thus, initial results from the Extension Project suggested that existing Ministry of Health and Family Planning staff density and work arrangements were insufficient for replicating the Matlab service model. Additional financial and staff resources would be needed to achieve similar results in Extension Project areas. Projections showed that implementing Matlab's fieldworker-to-population ratio within the national programme would require the hiring and deployment of at least 10 000 additional workers throughout Bangladesh (16). Other changes were required to institute the Matlab approach in government service areas, such as a unified health and family planning administrative system, and well-paid and highly committed supervisors. Research documenting the problems with the transfer of Matlab operations to Extension Project areas provided evidence that replicating Matlab was feasible if resources were mobilized for making the programme work.

This conclusion had direct bearing on a 1983 dialogue between the Ministry of Health and Family Planning and the World Bank about the contents of forthcoming loan agreements. Deliberations succeeded in mobilizing financial support from the five-year World Bank Third Population and Health Project for recruitment, training and deployment of 12 000 additional female workers as well as for other crucial elements of the Matlab approach that were missing in the national programme. Community workers were trained to provide injectable contraceptives at the doorstep, management information systems were reformed, and training was instituted to broaden the health service capabilities of family planning workers. Some structural features of the Matlab system were not scaled up, such as an integrated health and family planning supervisory system and target-free work assignments. Nonetheless, substantial Matlab-inspired operational changes were instituted, all of which were specified in detail in national planning documents and funded by a US$ 2 per capita per year credit from the World Bank agreement (17). Thus, research showing a lack of impact on the volume of service encounters, contraceptive use and health indicators of the initial Extension Project became a resource for mobilizing external funding for scaling up (18).

With the launching of the World Bank Third Population and Health Project, research priorities shifted from assessing Extension Project impact to generating evidence for guiding national reforms in training, supervision and management (13). The scaling-up process that ensued was driven by plans, policies, resources, directives and actions specified in the agreement between the Bangladesh Government and the World Bank. Each new ingredient, such as the procedures for recruiting additional fieldworkers as well as the implementation of doorstep provision of injectables, was first tested in the Extension area before being used more widely. The World Bank funded national policy conferences, newsletters and other activities for building momentum for change. Government directives were used to communicate evidence, progress and policies to all relevant health officials in the country. Evidence used in this communication process was based on Matlab research, studies of the replication effort in Extension Project areas, and national surveys for monitoring fertility and childhood mortality reduction trends. Findings from this monitoring programme showed that demographic transition over the period 1980–1995 ranked among the most rapid ever recorded, with patterns of variance consistent with the hypothesis that scaling up community-based services contributed to rapid demographic change (19, 20).

The Ghana case

In 1978, the International Conference on Primary Health Care convened in Alma-Ata, USSR (now Almaty, Kazakhstan) declared "Health for All" as a priority for all countries by the year 2000. Yet as the Millennium approached, poor access to primary health-care services explained much of the excess mortality and unwanted fertility throughout Africa. Ghana exemplifies the health-care accessibility problem. In the 1990s, 70% of the population resided in communities that were 8 km or more from the nearest health facility (21). In these areas, mortality was 40% higher and family planning use was considerably lower than in communities located closer to service points. Fertility and mortality remained high and unchanging, despite two decades of commitment to developing effective services.

In 1991, the Government of Ghana had launched a national community health programme in which volunteers were deployed to communities, and paid professional nurses were stationed at district and sub-district health centres. This community health programme reflected international advocacy for two strategies. One emphasized the potential value of community-based volunteer health services for extending affordable primary health care to all households. Advocates of volunteer programmes argued that vibrant social institutions for organizing daily life could be marshalled for organizing community-based management, financing and leadership of health services. Reliance on existing social institutions would reduce costs, sustain services and generate social acceptance of health and family planning services (22, 23). A contrasting strategy emphasized the value of existing clinical resources and the need to increase communities' access to professional health service providers. In this view, nurses could be trained and stationed in communities to offer a range of health interventions and technologies that volunteers would not be competent to provide. These two approaches were implemented on a national scale without carrying out research to guide operational planning.

Evaluations of the Ghana community health programme in the early 1990s showed that neither the volunteer approach nor community health nursing services were working. Volunteer turnover was high, supervision was lax and organizational deficiencies constrained programme progress. Nonetheless, reliance on volunteers remained an appealing policy option, since community deployment of professional workers appeared to require unsustainable investment in facilities, equipment and personnel (24). The Community Health Nurses programme also faced serious obstacles. By 1992, nearly 2000 nurses had been hired, trained for 18 months and posted to districts throughout Ghana. Because community facilities where nurses could work and live were lacking, however, the programme posted all nurses to sub-district health centres that were located over 10 km, on average, from the rural households they were serving. Communities were not connected with the initiative and contributed little to its sustainability. Case-loads were low and demographic indicators were not improving, bringing into question prospects that community nurse deployment could contribute to community health (25).

In response to the need for evidence to guide health policy, the Ministry of Health established a research centre in Navrongo Town of Kassena-Nankana District of the Upper East Region to investigate the causes and consequences of the health problems of northern Ghana (26). The economic, social and health circumstances of the study area paralleled conditions that prevailed in Matlab. Kassena-Nankana District is located in a remote, impoverished, traditional area where social norms sustain high fertility and impede progress with health interventions (27). Baseline mortality, and especially childhood mortality, in the locality was well above national levels. Contraceptive use was rare owing to complex social, gender and economic barriers to fertility regulation (27). The economy in the study area was dominated by subsistence agriculture and near-famine conditions each year; literacy was low (particularly among women); and traditions of marriage, kinship and family-building emphasized the economic and security value of large families. Health-care decision-making was strongly influenced by traditional beliefs, animist rites and poverty. Placing experimental research in such an unpromising locality ensured that any project success arising from interventions could not be dismissed as a byproduct of favourable trends and circumstances.

The Navrongo experiment was initially launched as a pilot project in 1994. The pilot was designed to avoid the potential pitfalls of importing an operational design inappropriate to local conditions, and of organizing a large and complex experiment which then fails. The pilot trial was conducted in three villages. Focus groups with local leaders, women of reproductive age, married men and community health nurses were convened to assess perceived health service needs and ways to alleviate known deficiencies of the national community health programme. These discussions clarified sustainable ways to engage communities in the construction of facilities that would end nurse isolation, support nurse operations, promote culturally acceptable means of providing family planning, and develop and sustain leadership. Focus group discussions were followed by posting nurses in the three pilot communities with the intent of launching community-based preventive, curative and referral health services. Follow-up focus groups gauged community and worker reactions to the pilot programme. Recommendations were used to modify implementation plans for training and deploying nurses, fostering volunteer support and sustaining community engagement with the programme (28).

After 18 months of the pilot trial and continued dialogue, an experimental study was launched in 1996 to assess the impact of these pilot strategies. The experimental phase used the two strategies corresponding to domains of the policy debate: one arm of the experiment tested the impact of mobilizing traditions to ensure sustainable volunteer participation in the programme and community involvement in supervising and managing volunteer operations. Chiefs, lineage heads and women's social networks were approached and then trained to build Community Health Compounds where nurses could be posted. Once this task was completed, this arm of the experiment focused on organizing the work of community health volunteers and building community participation for the management of their work.

The second arm of the experiment tested the impact of relocating nurses from sub-district clinics to community locations. Once nurses had been trained in community liaison methods and provided with motorbikes, basic drugs and primary health-care equipment, they were posted to Community Health Compounds where they offered vaccination services, treatment of common ailments (including malaria, acute respiratory infections and diarrhoeal diseases) and reproductive health and family planning services. Family planning options included the provision of injectable contraception, oral contraceptives and condoms in homes, and referral services for clinical methods, such as the five-year sub-dermal implant (29). Taken together, the two dimensions of the experiment comprised a four-cell design, since each dimension could be implemented independently, jointly or not at all (26). In the combined cell of the experiment, community liaison was directed to building community leadership of both volunteer and nurse service operations.

Early Navrongo research showed that relocating nurses to communities increased the service volume, family planning prevalence and immunization coverage, and expanded the range and quality of reproductive health care. Health services provided by a single nurse exceeded the typical case-load of a sub-district health centre. By 1999, district-wide experimental results showed that the total fertility rate had declined by one birth relative to comparison area levels; childhood mortality among 1–5-year-olds was reduced by over a third in the initial three project impact years that began in 1997 (30) and by two thirds by the end of 2003. Thus, the Navrongo project achieved the child survival Millennium Development Goal in six years (31, 32).

The Navrongo resource team presented its findings to senior Ministry of Health officials in early 1998, leading the Ministry to adopt the Navrongo model as the guide for community health services nationwide. To build consensus for this policy, in 1998 the first in a series of

National Health Forum conferences was convened for all 110 District Health Management Teams in Ghana. Key Navrongo results were presented and discussed in an open forum to elicit reactions from district and regional managers from all 10 regions, the heads of directorates responsible for planning, human resources, finance, public health and logistics, as well as the Minister and the Vice President of Ghana. Despite clear support from senior officials, responses from District Health Management Teams closely paralleled reactions to the Matlab experiment in Bangladesh: most of their discussion questioned the relevance of the Navrongo experiment for national policy on grounds that research stations have unique resources and capabilities that the typical district could not replicate. Debate about service strategies thus shifted from questions about the potential impact of the Navrongo model to new questions about the feasibility of replicating the approach in non-research settings.

Responding to this debate, the Ministry of Health arranged for national, regional and district officials to observe Navrongo operations first hand. These exchanges showed that experimental research was insufficient for building policy consensus, because Navrongo's unique resources were widely viewed as nonreplicable. A new phase of work was therefore needed in response to new policy questions about the replicability and sustainability of the Navrongo system.

In 1998, the Volta Regional Health Administration and the District Health Management Team from Nkwanta District took on this validation task and began by completing a six-week Navrongo field orientation on implementing and managing the model. The replication project in Nkwanta tested the means of establishing the Navrongo model services in two communities. Dialogue with community members produced advice on ways to adapt the model to local circumstances. Experience with this replication effort was carefully documented and presented at senior staff meetings and national health policy conferences.

Replication results from Nkwanta clarified mechanisms for implementing the Navrongo approach and established its credibility (33). Conferences convened to interpret the continuing research outcomes of Navrongo and the operational success of Nkwanta led to a 1999 decision to create the Community-based Health Planning and Services (CHPS) initiative, a national programme for fostering the scaling-up of the Navrongo community health service model. The policy initially focused on the need for "lead districts" in each of Ghana's 10 regions, where Navrongo-like services could be adapted to local realities and could then guide development of community-based care in neighbouring districts in the manner of replication and adaptation that Nkwanta had demonstrated. This new policy recognized the need to mobilize a process that would encourage the diffusion of innovation, demonstration and peer leadership at the local level. Attention focused on sustaining district-level implementation rather than developing a centrally directed operational plan.

As the scaling-up phase took hold, the value of sustaining experimental research for the duration of the process was demonstrated. To enhance Ministry of Health ownership of the project, the Navrongo resource team collaborated with senior officials of the Ministry on the use of results. Project protocol details were agreed upon prior to donor involvement. The Navrongo Centre reports to the Health Research Unit in Accra, which in turn reports to the Ghana Health Service's Policy Planning, Monitoring and Evaluation Division (PPMED). Its finances and staffing, however, are independent of the public sector bureaucracy, in order to maximize flexibility and leadership. The integration of Navrongo into the policy system facilitates links between Navrongo research dissemination activities and routine Ghana Health Service internal communication, conferences and meetings. Thus, Navrongo continues to contribute to scaling up by shifting its service operation from a district for an experimental trial to a field site for demonstration and counterpart training for District Health Management Teams.

Scaling-up activities outside of Navrongo and Nkwanta are stimulated and sustained through peer exchanges. District teams composed of two community nurses, their supervisor, the public health nurse and the Director of Medical Services are prepared to implement the programme after a 10-day orientation to routine community-based service work in Navrongo. Once redeployed to their home districts, teams develop community-based planning activities in one or two pilot zones. After strategic planning and trial, each team scales up operations within its respective district, according to the availability of staffing and resources (34). Navrongo and Nkwanta disseminate newsletters which report community reactions to project activities. Thus the experience of community participants contributes to the consensus among health officers in Ghana that going to scale is feasible and desirable. Scaling up is therefore highly decentralized and peer directed.

Despite the focus on decentralization and peer leadership, scaling up in Ghana has had strong commitment from the central government. The programme has experienced operational problems and delays that have required policy responses and directives (for a discussion, see 29, 34). While there have been problems, by the end of 2005 scaling-up activities had been launched in all of the 110 districts of Ghana and full implementation of the programme was underway in 20 districts.

A shared model for evidence-based reform

The sequence of actions, changing generations of questions, and roles of research in Bangladesh and Ghana followed a common evidence-based reform process in four phases.

Phase 1: participatory planning

Beginning with the question, "What type of services are appropriate?" a Phase 1 programme of adaptive development of strategies was used to configure a service model with operational details that were informed by continuous evaluation and participatory planning. In Matlab, the failed Contraceptive Distribution Project provided the focus for participatory qualitative appraisal of the reasons for failure and implications for configuring a follow-on experiment. In Navrongo, participatory pilot appraisal provided a similar function. Participatory planning represents a tool of "open systems" organizational development: social institutions, traditions and organizational norms are tapped to improve the efficiency and functioning of formal organizations (35).

Phase 2: factorial trial

Matlab and Navrongo had advanced institutional capabilities for conducting vaccine trials and epidemiological research. Just as health technologies could be evaluated, community health service systems could be tested, with health and demographic outcomes as the variables of interest. Experimental research provided credible evidence that the approaches tested actually helped the population served. Putting debate to rest was crucial to health reform. Both Matlab and Navrongo provided definitive evidence that if services were designed to be sensitive to women's needs they would lead to increased contraceptive prevalence, greater satisfaction and fertility decline as well as improved child survival. These results could be achieved with affordable and simple procedures for reaching families in need.

Phase 3: validation research

The scientific rigour of Matlab and Navrongo required advanced scientific capabilities that were complex and expensive to manage. The greater the rigour of trials, the greater the tendency of researchers to isolate operations from the user system and to deploy resources that are difficult to replicate. The penchant for elegant research designs sometimes precipitates questions about the "Hawthorne effect" – reference to a classic study showing that results were related more to the effect of being observed than to the intervention under trial (36). More recently, this term is applied to research conducted with non-replicable human and financial resources. Disproving the Hawthorne effect requires unobtrusive and low-cost research on the replicability of experimental findings and the sustainability of the scaling-up process (14, 33). Therefore, in both Bangladesh and Ghana, a beyond-the-experiment phase was launched to bridge the gap between field trials and large-scale programmes by shifting research from questions about the health and demographic impact of operations to questions about the feasibility and sustainability of innovations in non-research settings.

Phase 4: monitoring the scaling-up process

The dissemination of credible evidence of project impact on fertility and mortality, and validation that service innovations could be replicated under normal programme conditions, motivated decisions to scale up operations. In Ghana, the process is still emerging and its national demographic impact is unknown, but research systems permit continuous appraisal of the pace, coverage and content of operational change. In Bangladesh, research shifted from impact assessment to monitoring the change process as a component activity of the World Bank's lending agreement that funded scaling up. In both settings, research provided evidence on whether scaling up was occurring, what was working well and what required change. Thus, as scaling up accelerated, the questions guiding research shifted from feasibility and consensus building to the challenge of refining the scaling-up process.

Adapting scaling-up strategies to contrasting settings

Common features of projects that foster the utilization of research for national policy and programme development are well known (37–42). Less is known about ways in which scaling-up efforts in contrasting settings should differ. The Bangladesh and Ghana cases demonstrate that the effective utilization of evidence in contrasting settings generates divergent scaling-up strategies.

Social organization

While the two countries are predominantly agrarian and share similar levels of economic development, they have markedly different patterns of social organization and land tenure customs. Although Bangladesh is rapidly urbanizing, until recently it was a peasant society in which economic opportunity is linked to inherited social status. Ghana, by contrast, is an ethnically diverse society in which land is communal and held in trust by chiefs, and economic opportunity is less linked to inheritance than to achievement that derives from individual effort facilitated by kindred, clan or ethnic network affiliation. In the Bangladesh case, the Bengali homogeneity of society permits a degree of centralization and standardization of scaling-up policy that would be dysfunctional in the heterogeneous Ghanaian societal context. Organizing collective action and communication through kindred groups is facilitated by Ghanaian social institutions, provided that actual organizing activities are adapted to local tradition. Collective community action strategies are less compatible with Bangladeshi society, and strategic adaptation is less essential than in Ghana.

Leadership traditions

Community leadership and social structure is well defined in Ghana, and village governance is associated with traditions that define roles in decision-making, consensus-building and collective action. Bangladeshi community governance is less structured and relatively diffuse. Leadership and authority are defined by wealth and patronage derived from land holding, relative economic standing, power alliances and ad hoc social networks that lack permanence across generations or predictability across localities. In Bangladesh, community organization was relatively less important to the scaling-up process than was the case in Ghana, where the spread of community health services has been a natural product of local traditions of communication and collective action. Gatherings, networks and other traditions that foster exchanges among communities and groups also have disseminated the benefits of community services in implementing districts. In this manner, communication traditions amplified the spontaneous diffusion of Navrongo innovations. Such mechanisms were relatively unimportant in Bangladesh.

Because scaling-up design in these settings was the product of locally gathered evidence on how best to proceed, societal differences led programme planners to pursue different strategies for organizational development. For example, social organization is diffuse in Bangladesh but relatively structured in Ghana. Community organizational resources were therefore a minor component of the scaling-up strategy in Bangladesh, but a major factor in Ghana. Sustaining the change process in Bangladesh depended upon continued commitment of external, top-down bureaucratic processes. The change process is more appropriately instituted in Ghana as lateral networks for spreading consensus through the diffusion of social support for innovation. In Bangladesh, volunteerism is more difficult to implement and sustain than in Ghana, where corporate community values are engrained and vibrant, and volunteer accountability to community leaders is socially grounded.

Leadership in Bangladesh is more likely to emerge from formal organizations than community institutions; in Ghana, organizational change derives from grassroots partnerships between traditional leaders, politicians and health professionals. While establishing such partnerships is challenging, it is sustainable with minimal external investment once the health system engages traditional leaders in respectful and culturally appropriate ways. In contrast, instilling leadership for sustaining change in Bangladesh is relatively dependent upon external resources, government orders or rank in the civil bureaucracy.

Scaling up in Ghana spreads by peer demonstration, diffusion and teamwork rather than by central order and fiat. Moreover, in the multicultural context of Ghana, adapting strategies to local conditions is more important than in Bangladesh, where national models are likely to have more relevance owing to the uniform cultural context. Therefore, in Ghana, strategies for decentralization have a prominent role in scaling up; whereas in Bangladesh, scaling up has been a relatively centralized function of the national programme.

Bureaucratic traditions

Other institutional contrasts had major effects on generating contrasting approaches to scaling up. The institutional histories of public sector organizations in Bangladesh and Ghana vary in ways that explain differences between their scaling-up programmes. In the colonial era, British India – which included areas that now constitute Bangladesh – was administered through direct control of the civil bureaucracy. Even in the Pakistan era, the public bureaucracy was externally controlled, with well-articulated mechanisms for the promulgation of top-down directives, narrow spans of authority and limited scope for decentralization. By contrast, civil bureaucracy is a relatively recent historical development in Ghana. British colonial rule was indirect, allowing traditional authorities to retain their customary powers, de-emphasizing the authority of the central bureaucracy by maintaining order through traditional governance of communities. Thus, a Bangladeshi villager in the British era routinely interacted with district representatives from ministries responsible for agriculture, education, health and public order. In contrast, a Ghanaian villager seeking to resolve a dispute in the colonial era would turn to a native court or a chieftaincy council, led by a traditional authority figure, to resolve minor disputes and grievances or launch community dialogue about all matters of collective interest. In this manner, local traditional communication and governance systems were sustained by colonial authorities, providing historical grounding for decentralization in Ghana and not in Bangladesh.

Features of the institutional legacy of large-scale organizations, combined with the contrasting social environments, define fundamentally different contexts for scaling up programmes. Of these, the most prominent difference between the Bangladesh and Ghana case-studies is the relative importance of the diffusion of innovation versus planned organizational change. In Bangladesh, planned organizational change and formal orders have played a more important role in scaling up than the spontaneous diffusion of innovation at the district level.

The role of external resources

The contrasting revenue circumstances of Bangladesh and Ghana scaling-up examples amplify these contrasts. In Bangladesh, demonstration of the Matlab system in two replication sites was followed by official pursuit of donor resources for the incremental costs of large-scale programmatic change. Earmarked World Bank funding permitted officials to plan and finance the expansion of hiring, construction and worker training. Training, in turn, was focused on developing front-line worker technical skills rather than competency in community mobilization. Although community work was essential to the Bangladesh programme, and doorstep services were crucial to its success, instituting change to that end was less a grassroots effort than a top-down bureaucratic initiative financed from afar. Clinics, salaries, pharmaceutical costs and other resources were line items in national budgets that were heavily financed by the World Bank and other donors. Thus, even without local political engagement or grass-roots mobilization, the Bangladesh scaling-up programme worked.

In contrast, Ghana has relied less on international resources than on local financing and community resource leveraging. This has slowed implementation because incremental resources for essential drugs, equipment and staff are lacking. Where the CHPS initiative has worked well in Ghana, demonstration of the community-based model in pilot areas has led neighbouring communities to press district authorities for local resources to finance programme expansion. This process has an element of guided direction, however. A national training programme has developed staff capacity for implementation, focusing resources on training supervisors in community mobilization and other activities that are needed for sustaining the scaling-up process. However, while these national activities are crucial, community-based health care has been developed mainly through locally tailored and indigenously funded adaptations of the Navrongo service system that emerge from district pilot trials. Rather than providing a rigid blueprint for districts to replicate, Navrongo and Nkwanta demonstration activities are designed to catalyse the process of operational change, providing visiting teams with general ideas that require local testing, adaptation and trial. Scaling up depends upon local resources, volunteerism and district assembly commitment. Success required more initiative and leadership at the periphery than was the case in Bangladesh (34, 43).

In Ghana, dependence on local resources was a matter of necessity rather than design, however. External assistance for health is merged with Government of Ghana revenue through health sector reform policies that are collectively termed the sector-wide approach. World Bank and European funding of this approach is extensive, but revenue for the health sector is planned as a common fund. Scaling up in Ghana has had no independent budget line for incremental costs, or donor earmarking of revenue for specific components of the programme. Foreign assistance has been directed to sustaining external technical support for CHPS training, communication and research activities rather than revenue for financing the direct costs of implementation. As a result, progress with scaling up in Ghana has been much slower than was the case in Bangladesh, where revenue was earmarked for direct programme costs. Thus, scaling up in Ghana depends upon financing and priority setting that is integrated into the general administrative processes of the Ghana Health Service; external support for the current overall health revenue budget is about half the level of funding provided to the health sector in Bangladesh in the 1980s and 1990s. Ghana has been forced by circumstances to sustain its programme with less external backing and greater reliance on community support.

Conclusion

The examples reviewed in this chapter are relevant to the organizational development needs of health programmes in the world's poorest regions. Their experience indicates that problems impeding programme reform and development can be surmounted and that large public programmes can be guided by research, even in resource-constrained settings. The Bangladesh and Ghana examples attest to the importance of integrating research into the process of scaling up that begins with the development and testing of innovations and proceeds to expansion of successful pilot and/or experimental projects. This is preferable to conducting research as a stand-alone activity to be utilized and scaled up as an afterthought. While adopting international best practices for designing national reforms, strategies must not be isolated from social and institutional realities, which must form the basis for policy and programme development. Overly internationalizing programme strategy, without guidance from locally grounded research, can isolate plans from social and institutional reality, fostering top-down planning when practical bottom-up guidance is badly needed. As the Bangladesh and Ghana cases demonstrate, the content, change process and scaled-up programme can be adapted to the local context. This process of adaptation benefits from the integration of research into the organizational reform programme.

New health technologies are often proposed as the answer to problems when, in fact, it is a malaise of the service system that deprives families of access to technologies. Projects in Bangladesh and Ghana demonstrate an approach to organizational development that addresses the need for strategies to improve programme performance. The initiatives succeeded not because they followed a common agenda for scaling up. They succeeded because similar research approaches steered the development of the innovative service packages and the scaling-up agenda in ways that adapted directions to indigenous realities and needs. Their success demonstrates that large-scale organizational change in reproductive and child health programmes is neither impossible nor unaffordable in resource-constrained settings.

Acknowledgements

This paper was made possible through support provided by the Office of Population, Bureau for Global Programs, Field Support and Research, of the United States Agency for International Development, under the terms of Award No. HRN-A-00-99-00010. The opinions expressed herein are those of the authors and do not necessarily reflect the views of the United States Agency for International Development.

References

1. Gwatkin DR. How well do health programmes reach the poor? *The Lancet*, 2003, 361:540–541.

2. Rowe AK, de Savigny D, Lanata CF et al. How can we achieve and maintain high-quality performance of health workers in low-resource settings? *The Lancet*, 2005, 366:1026–1035.

3. Curlin GT, Hossain B, Chen LC. Demographic crisis: the impact of the Bangladesh Independence War (1971) on births and deaths in a rural area of Bangladesh. *Population Studies*, 1976, 30:87–105.

4. Mosley WH, Chen LC. An analytical framework for the study of child survival in developing countries. *Population and Development Review*, 1984, 10:25–48.

5. Arthur WB, McNicoll G. An analytical survey of population and development in Bangladesh. *Population and Development Review*, 1978, 4:23–80.

6.   Cain M. Risk, fertility, and family planning in a Bangladesh village. *Studies in Family Planning*, 1980, 11:219–223.

7.   Demeny P. Observations on population policy and population programme in Bangladesh. *Population and Development Review*, 1975, 1:307–321.

8.   Aziz KMA, Mosley HW. The history, methodology and main findings of the Matlab project in Bangladesh. In: Das Gupta M et al., eds. *Prospective community studies in developing countries*. Oxford, University of Oxford Press, 1997:28–53.

9.   Stinson WS, Phillips JF, Rahman M et al. The demographic impact of the contraceptive distribution project in Matlab, Bangladesh. *Studies in Family Planning*, 1982, 13:141–148.

10.   Bhatia S, Mosley WH, Faruque ASG et al. The Matlab Family Planning Health Services Project. *Studies in Family Planning*, 1980, 11:202–212.

11.   Phillips JF, Simmons R, Koenig MA et al. The determinants of reproductive change in a traditional society: evidence from Matlab, Bangladesh. *Studies in Family Planning*, 1988, 19:313–334.

12.   LeGrand TK, Phillips JF. The effect of fertility reductions on infant and child mortality: evidence from Matlab in rural Bangladesh. *Population Studies*, 1996, 50:51–68.

13.   Phillips JF. Translating pilot project success into national policy development: the Matlab and MCH-FP extension projects in Bangladesh. In: Halstead SB, Walsh JA, eds. *Why things work: case histories in development*. Boston, MA, Adams Publishing Group, 1990:19–38.

14.   Phillips JF, Simmons R, Simmons G et al. Transferring health and family planning service innovations to the public sector: an experiment in organization development in Bangladesh. *Studies in Family Planning*, 1984, 15:62–73.

15.   Hossain MB, Phillips JF. The impact of outreach on the continuity of contraceptive use in rural Bangladesh. *Studies in Family Planning*, 1996, 27:98–106.

16.   Simmons R, Baqee L, Koenig MA et al. Beyond supply: the institutional potential of female family planning workers in rural Bangladesh. *Studies in Family Planning*, 1988, 19:29–38.

17.   Buse K, Gwin C. The World Bank and global cooperation in health: the case of Bangladesh. *The Lancet*, 1998, 351:665–669.

18.   Haaga J, Maru R. The effect of operations research on program changes in Bangladesh. *Studies in Family Planning*, 1996, 27:76–87.

19. Cleland J, Phillips JF, Amin S. *The determinants of reproductive change in Bangladesh: success in a challenging environment*. Washington, DC, The World Bank, 1994.

20. Phillips JF, Hossain MB, Arends-Kuenning M. The long-term demographic role of community-based family planning in rural Bangladesh. *Studies in Family Planning*, 1996, 27: 204–219.

21. *A profile of health inequities in Ghana*. Accra, Ministry of Health of the Republic of Ghana, 1998.

22. Knippenberg R, Levy-Bruhl D, Osseni R et al. *The Bamako Initiative: primary health care*. New York, United Nations Children's Fund, 1990.

23. *The Bamako Initiative: a progress report*. New York, United Nations Children's Fund, 1991 (unpublished monograph).

24. Adjei S, Senah K, Cofie P. *Study on the implications of community health workers' distributing drugs in Ghana*. Accra, Ministry of Health of the Republic of Ghana, 1995 (Health Research Unit, unpublished).

25. Agyepong IA, Marfo C. *Is there a place for community-based health workers in primary health care delivery in Ghana? Internal evaluation of the Dangme West District Village Health Worker Programme*. Accra, Ministry of Health of the Republic of Ghana, 1992 (Health Research Unit, unpublished).

26. Binka FN, Nazzar A, Phillips JF. The Navrongo community health and family planning project. *Studies in Family Planning*, 1995, 26:121–139.

27. Adongo PB, Phillips JF, Kajihara BZ et al. Cultural factors constraining the introduction of family planning among the Kassena-Nankana of northern Ghana. *Social Science and Medicine*, 1997, 45:1789–1804.

28. Nazzar A, Adongo PB, Binka F et al. Involving a traditional community in strategic planning: the Navrongo community health and family planning project pilot study. *Studies in Family Planning*, 1995, 26:307–324.

29. Nyonator FK, Awoonor-Williams JK, Phillips JF et al. The Ghana community-based health planning and services initiative: fostering evidence-based organizational change and development in a resource-constrained setting. *Health Policy and Planning*, 2005, 20:25–34.

30. Pence BW, Nyarko P, Phillips JF et al. *The effect of community nurses and health volunteers on child mortality: the Navrongo community health and family planning project*. New York, The Population Council, 2005 (Policy Research Division Working Paper 200).

31. Binka FN, Bawah AA, Phillips JF et al. *Rapid achievement of the child survival Millennium Development Goal: evidence from the Navrongo experiment in northern Ghana.* 2005 (unpublished manuscript).

32. Phillips JF, Bawah AA, Binka FN. *The design, impact and utilization of the Navrongo experiment in Ghana.* New York, The Population Council, 2005 (Policy Research Division Working Paper 208).

33. Awoonor-Williams JK, Feinglass ES, Tobey R et al. Bridging the gap between evidence-based innovation and national health sector reform in Ghana. *Studies in Family Planning*, 2004, 35:161–177.

34. Nyonator FK, Jones TC, Miller RA et al. Guiding the Ghana Community-based Health Planning and Services approach to scaling up with qualitative systems appraisal. *International Quarterly of Community Health Education*, 2005, 23:189–213.

35. Katz D, Kahn RL, Adams JS. *The study of organizations.* San Francisco, CA, Jossey-Bass Inc., 1980.

36. Roethlisberger FJ, Dickson WJ. *Management and the workers.* Cambridge, MA, Harvard University Press, 1939.

37. Havelock R. *What do we know from research about the process of research utilization?* Paper presented at: International Conference on Making Population/Family Planning Research Useful, the communicators' contribution, Honolulu, 3–7 December 1978. Hawaii, East-West Communication Institute, 1979.

38. Cernada GP. *Knowledge into action: a guide to research utilization.* Farmingdale, NY, Baywood Publishing Company Inc., 1982.

39. Glaser EM, Abelson HH, Garrison KN. *Putting knowledge to use: facilitating the diffusion of knowledge and the implementation of planned change.* San Francisco, CA, Jossey-Bass Inc., 1983.

40. Davis P, Howden-Chapman P. Translating research findings into health policy. *Social Science and Medicine*, 1996, 43:865–872.

41. Bertrand J, Marin C. *Operations research: measuring its impact on service delivery and policy.* Baltimore, MD, Johns Hopkins University School of Public Health, 2001 (unpublished).

42. Simmons R, Brown J, Díaz M. Facilitating large-scale transitions to quality of care: an idea whose time has come. *Studies in Family Planning*, 2002, 33:61–75.

43.   Nyonator F, Phillips JF, Awoonor-Williams JK et al. *The impact of district partnering on scaling up community-based health sector reform in Ghana.* Paper presented at: Annual Conference of the Global Health Council, Washington, DC, 31 May–3 June 2005.

Chapter 7

Scaling up family planning service innovations in Brazil: the influence of politics and decentralization

Juan Díaz, Ruth Simmons, Margarita Díaz, Francisco Cabral, Magda Chinaglia[a]

Summary

The principles of strategic management suggest that a major step in ensuring effective scaling up is to understand the diverse environments in which health service innovations are expanded. When service innovations are expanded in the public sector, the political and administrative institutions, as well as the health sector setting constitute major environmental influences. This chapter analyses these factors in Brazil, using the experience of a project which sought to enhance equitable access and improve the quality of care in public sector family planning services. Nongovernmental organizations acted as the resource team that facilitated the testing of the original service innovations in one municipality and then assisted with their expansion to others. The chapter shows that scaling up is influenced by an ongoing process of decentralization and by the politics of family planning. Scaling up family planning innovations faces special challenges, which would not be encountered in other areas of reproductive health in Brazil.

Introduction

The principles of strategic management suggest that a major step in ensuring effective scaling up is to understand the diverse environments in which health service innovations are expanded (1). These environments, or contexts, shape the opportunities and constraints that proponents of scaling up must navigate (see Chapter 1). When service innovations are expanded in the public sector, the political and administrative institutions, as well as the health sector setting constitute major environmental influences. This chapter analyses these factors

---

[a] The authors of this chapter are members of the nongovernmental team that facilitated the scaling up of reproductive health services in the public sector. They belong to the following institutions: Reprolatina (a Brazilian nongovernmental organization), the Population Council office of Brazil and the University of Michigan.

in Brazil, using the experience of a project which sought to enhance equitable access and improve the quality of public sector family planning services. Nongovernmental organizations (NGOs) acted as the resource team that facilitated the testing of the original service innovations in one municipality and then assisted with their expansion to others. We show that scaling up is influenced by an ongoing process of decentralization and by the politics of family planning. Scaling up family planning innovations in Brazil faces special challenges that would not be encountered in other areas of reproductive health.

In Brazil, an estimated 75% of the population depend on the public sector for their health care (2), which at the primary level is provided through health posts, health centres or community-based family health outreach services (3). Clinic-based family planning services are provided by gynaecologists, assisted by auxiliary and technical nursing personnel, on contract with the public sector for a specified number of hours. These services are free of charge to the users. The community-based family health service is supposed to include contraceptive care, but lack of contraceptive supplies is a major barrier. The Sociedad Civil Bem-Estar Familiar, an NGO, has provided extensive support to the public sector family planning programme, maintaining agreements with 1001 municipalities predominantly in the north-east of the country for the provision of technical assistance, training and evaluation (4). Although public sector responsibilities have been established and some services are indeed available, overall access to family planning care is extremely constrained and the care that is provided tends to be of poor quality (5–7).

In 1995 a project in the municipality of Santa Barbara d'Oeste (referred to in this chapter as Santa Barbara) in the State of São Paulo in southern Brazil initiated a systematic process of dealing with these weaknesses in access and quality of care. Interventions in the pilot municipality focused on:

- upgrading all elements of quality of care through training;
- restructuring providers' roles and service delivery patterns so as to maximize the use of scarce medical personnel;
- improving the management process in order to ensure accountability and supportive supervision;
- creating a referral centre where regular availability of contraceptive care would be assured;
- establishing a participatory process including representation from the community (8);
- introducing outpatient vasectomy services (9);
- developing a programme for adolescents.

Comprehensive training played a major role in introducing these innovations. In 1997, evaluation results demonstrated that the public sector service system had improved availability, access, and the quality of family planning services within the resource constraints of the municipal health sector (10). Support from the NGO resource team of action researchers and trainers was an important factor in this success.

For most projects this would be the end of the story; but not so in this case. Activities in Santa Barbara were implemented as part of the Strategic Approach to Strengthening Reproductive Health Policies and Programmes sponsored by the World Health Organization (WHO) (11–13). One of the special characteristics of the Strategic Approach is its emphasis on scaling up (14). The positive evaluation results therefore raised the question whether the model implemented in the pilot, and the many lessons that were learned, could benefit other municipalities in Brazil. The resource team that had facilitated the development, implementation and evaluation of the project in Santa Barbara took on the challenge and, with funding from WHO, initiated and supported replication of the approach in three other municipalities between 1997 and 1999.

Because their needs were similar, the three new municipalities adopted many of the core service innovations from Santa Barbara. In 1999, after three years of replication in these localities, significant improvements in access to services and their quality had once again been achieved. In fact, the process had been easier and faster because of the learning that had occurred in the pilot project (15). Santa Barbara was used as a demonstration site where professionals from the new municipalities could see how the innovations functioned in actual practice. Moreover, the NGO resource team was now more skilled in supporting the introduction of service innovations because of its experience in the pilot site which resulted in greater sophistication in navigating health sector and local government institutions.

This scaling-up success, however, posed a dilemma as well as a new question. Brazil has over 5500 municipalities, but the project had worked in only four. That scaling up would not proceed spontaneously, but instead requires active support from a resource team, became apparent during the first phase of expansion. In a decentralized health system such as Brazil this implies that a large number of local governments, whose management capacity tends to be weak, depend on external assistance in the process of adopting service innovations (16–18). The need and actual interest among municipalities in joining the project was great. In fact, the demand for such support during the first phase of expansion was more than what the resource team could offer.

For example, in one of the new municipalities, health professionals expressed disappointment that the level of support received had been less than they would have liked. Thus the question was whether the relatively small, nongovernmental team of action researchers and trainers could facilitate the process of expansion beyond what had been accomplished during the first phase of scaling up.

In 1999, funding from the Bill and Melinda Gates Foundation made it possible to continue the process of scaling up, and provided the opportunity to develop a strategy for multiplying the capacity to support expansion of service innovations. This strategy, implemented through what was now referred to as the Reprolatina Project, had two key components.

- Development of training capacity that would enable newly trained municipal trainers to expand training to all health posts and centres within their municipality and beyond. Creating a municipal resource team rather than relying exclusively on external facilitators would make it possible for local trainers to introduce innovations within their own municipality and subsequently expand them to neighbouring ones.

- Active networking and the use of information technology to facilitate information exchange and ensure that municipal innovators would support each other rather than rely exclusively on the NGO resource team.

Over the past six years, training capacity has been created in nine municipalities which, in turn, have expanded activities to an additional 26 smaller ones. Periodic participatory seminars for leaders of the municipal implementation teams and the creation of web-based conferences and other forms of electronic communications have enabled ongoing opportunities for experience sharing and social learning. Simultaneously the project has further refined its strategy for adolescents and training for local leaders. A discussion of the Reprolatina training approach is provided in the next chapter.

Many lessons have been learned in the course of scaling up. The one initially most underestimated is the importance of understanding the political, administrative and health sector contexts.[1] Throughout the project, this lesson has emerged as more and more important. At the beginning, the external resource team members were confident that they knew a great deal about the sociocultural, institutional and

---

[1] For a systematic assessment of the influence of social organization and political culture on decentralized health care in Brazil see *19*.

political environment of public sector family planning services. Certainly, enough was known about the health system and the bureaucratic institutions in Brazil to proceed with appropriate intervention strategies. Several years after seeking to expand service innovations to new municipalities, however, it is clear that learning about the institutional setting and about political culture never stops. More important still, learning must be actively encouraged, both among members of the resource team and among municipal partners. The public health system always holds surprises, especially since it continues to evolve and is highly variable among municipalities. In Brazil, where decentralization has become a major component of political and health sector reform, efforts to improve family planning and related services benefit from strategies that adjust to such ongoing change and variability.

This chapter identifies both environmental opportunities and constraints that affect the wider use of successfully tested programme innovations. In the Brazilian context, as in many others, the constraints can be daunting, but recognizing them should not discourage initiatives. Rather, taking constraints into account allows the innovators to choose realistic strategies, anticipate the level of resources needed, and assess the type, pace and extent of scale that can be achieved.

The information contained in this chapter comes from six sources: 1) participant observation, covering more than 10 years during which members of the resource team implemented the WHO-sponsored Strategic Approach and the Reprolatina Project; 2) published papers and unpublished reports from these projects; 3) qualitative assessments conducted in participating municipalities as a central component of the health service renewal process; 4) meetings and interviews with Ministry of Health, state and municipal officials; 5) official reports, laws and guidelines of the Ministry of Health; and 6) literature on health sector reform and decentralization in Brazil.

Decentralization: opportunities and constraints in scaling up

In Brazil, health reform began in the 1970s as part of a wider movement for the democratization of the country (20–23). The health reform movement advocated for the principles of universality and equality in health, seeking to combat the injustices of a bifurcated medical/healthcare system. Services were available through insurance programmes to workers in the formal sector of the economy, leaving the rural and urban poor without access to health care. Insurance programmes for workers were administered by the Instituto Nacional de Assistência Médica da Previdência Social (INAMPS, National Institute of Medical Care of the Social Welfare System) under the authority of the Ministry of Social Security;[2] other areas of health were the responsibility of the Ministry of Health. With return to democracy in 1984 many of the principles of the health reform movement were enshrined in article 196 of the Constitution (1988), which guarantees health as a universal right and commits the country to the provision of equal and universal access to services. Family planning is considered a basic right and the state is charged with the responsibility of providing educational and scientific resources to ensure access to care. Decentralization and the participation of civil society in policy development and implementation are mandated. The Constitution also declares that health services should be organized under a single, decentralized system, with a preventive focus and the participation of communities. With the formal creation of the Sistema Único de Saúde (SUS, Unified Health System), in 1990 (25), the dual authority over health was ended and the Ministry of Health assumed sole responsibility for public sector health care.

Decentralization in the health sector was formally initiated with the Basic Operating Rules of 1991, 1993 and 1996, by progressively shifting authority for decision-making to government at the state and municipal levels with major responsibility to the latter (21, 26). Such "municipalization" proceeds through transference of resources according to the capacity of the municipality to assume "full management of basic care"[3] or "full management of the municipal system".[4] In 2005, 88.2% of the 5561 municipalities in Brazil were still in the first stage of decentralization (28, 29).

Decentralization dictates a focus on horizontal scaling up

A distinction has been made in the literature between replication or expansion of innovations, and political, policy or legal scaling up (30, 31 and Chapter 1). The former is focused on geographical expansion or horizontal scaling up, and the latter on institutionalization or vertical scaling up.

---

[2] INAMPS was an autonomous institution associated with the Ministry of Social Security until 1990 when it became part of the Ministry of Health; it ceased to exist in 2002 (24).

[3] Municipalities with the "full management of basic care" receive a fixed per capita amount and, with these funds have to develop all primary health activities, including assistance and rehabilitation, prevention and health promotion. In addition, municipalities receive a variable amount for epidemiological surveillance, the environment, essential treatments, the family health programme and prevention of nutritional deficiencies.

[4] Municipalities with "full management of the municipal system" have more managerial autonomy and must provide primary, secondary and tertiary levels of care, including hospitalization. Where official agreements among municipalities have been made, they should also provide care to people referred from surrounding municipalities (27). These municipalities receive, besides the Piso de Atenção Básica (minimum level of services in primary care), resources for secondary and tertiary care, including some funds for specific programmes (26).

The process of decentralization in Brazil had major implications for the design of the pilot project in Santa Barbara and for subsequent scaling-up initiatives. It was clear from the outset that, given the municipalities' predominant role in programmatic decision-making, the focus would have to be on the municipality and that scaling up would have to proceed mainly as a process of geographical expansion. As we indicate below, this approach had advantages but also faced major constraints. Municipal autonomy facilitates the introduction of innovations, but sustainability and collaboration among municipalities in their expansion can be problematic.

Municipal autonomy facilitates the introduction of innovations

Municipal autonomy implies that local health authorities are able to institute major programmatic innovations as long as they comply with national policies and guidelines. These fully endorse, and in fact mandate, the provision of reproductive health services, including family planning (32–34). There is no need to obtain authorization from the state or federal level, or to provide information about what changes are being made. Thus, where municipal authorities are supportive, major service renewal can be initiated. Moreover, given the considerable fiscal discretion associated with decentralization, it is often possible to identify necessary local resources to improve facilities, ensure supplies or recruit additional staff.

In the pilot site, municipal autonomy was a clear advantage at the beginning of the project. The municipal health secretary was highly motivated to improve family planning services, and had turned to the nongovernmental resource team to provide training and other technical support (10). Local resources were mobilized to recruit additional health-care providers, to remodel one of the facilities to create a reproductive health referral centre, and to introduce an adolescent programme and a vasectomy service. This pattern repeated itself in the other municipalities (15). Federal or state regulations have not been an obstacle in the effort to expand innovations.

Politicization of technical issues and leadership changes threaten sustainability

Decentralization of authority to the municipal level has been associated with a change in the status of technical personnel which has had a negative effect on sustainability. Under the earlier centralized system, health professionals had more autonomy to make decisions because they were employed by the federal government rather than by the municipality (25). As part of a competitively recruited cadre of federal appointees in permanent positions, they also had greater job security. Personnel hired at the municipal level, in contrast, often do not have secure jobs. Facing severe and regular financial constraints, local legislatures tend to be unwilling to authorize permanent positions that require competitive recruitment. As a consequence, most recruitment is for jobs on temporary contracts from which staff can be easily dismissed. This has made technical professionals subject to greater political accountability and has led to frequent changes among key personnel.

Such turnover generally occurs in the wake of elections, especially when the party in power changes, but it also takes place at other times. In the period between the last two local elections, project municipalities changed their secretary of health several times, with an average of three replacements between 2000 and 2004; one municipality had seven. Leadership change tends to be associated with replacement of other staff who are political appointees or personal friends. For example, the coordinators of the Women's Health Programme – who play a central role in implementing reproductive health service innovations – were always removed at the same time as the health secretary. Frequent personnel change has undermined the sustainability of health service innovations and has required extensive resource-team support to ensure continuity.

The impact of leadership change is exacerbated by the fact that new officials are rarely briefed about ongoing programmes and often come with specific instructions to abandon innovations in order to weaken the political image of the previous administration (35). Given the autonomy of elected municipal officials, innovations can be abolished by a new administration even though they are fully integrated into local service systems. Even when the party in power is confirmed by the election, a change of the mayor may require several months to reinitiate activities with new authorities. As a result, the window of opportunity for building new initiatives lasts at best four years, and the sustainability of innovations, no matter how beneficial, is not easily ensured.

Lack of collaboration between municipalities jeopardizes scaling up

The federally mandated pattern of decentralization officially encourages collaboration among municipalities (36) which could increase access to needed technology for more people and could provide a mechanism for scaling up health service innovations. In reality, however, political and financial considerations discouraged such collaboration, thereby curtailing opportunities for scaling up. In the experience of the Reprolatina Project, collaboration was not easily realized for using newly trained reproductive health trainers to train neighbouring municipalities. Some health and local authorities saw collaboration as a beneficial strategy, arguing that improved capacity in neighbouring municipalities would reduce the number of patients who crossed municipal borders to seek care in their health facilities. Others, however, objected to such training as an unjustified use of municipal resources for neighbouring areas. Political rivalries among office-holders from different parties added to the difficulties of arriving at collaborative agreements.

As a result of these constraints, efforts to utilize newly created training capacity as a means of expanding innovations to neighbouring municipalities did not always succeed. A collaborative strategy for scaling up health service innovations among municipalities was thus not as powerful a tool as expected. Multiplying training capacity improved the ability of project municipalities to respond to training needs within the municipality but continued to require heavy reliance on the training role of the project's core resource team in the expansion to other municipalities.

Limited opportunities for vertical scaling up in a decentralized setting

Scaling up should involve not only the expansion of innovations from site to site but also interventions at the political, policy and legal levels – which has been defined as vertical scaling up (30). Such interventions are essential for all levels of government but are particularly critical for higher echelons. Institutionalization at these levels facilitates and sustains the process of expansion. Effective decentralization – and by implication effective scaling up – requires a strong level of intergovernmental liaison and some oversight or incentives from the state and federal level (21).

Even though much decision-making authority passes to the municipality in the process of decentralization in Brazil, the federal and state government maintains critical functions which can and should be engaged in scaling up. Federal-level initiatives occur in regard to the provision of contraceptive supplies to municipalities and in priority setting through the creation of financial incentives for special programmes. The state level plays a role in the allocation of resources for training. If scaling-up advocates succeed in influencing decisions in these areas, the prospects for institutionalizing and expanding innovations are substantially enhanced. The Reprolatina Project attempted to work on the vertical scaling up, but the overall success in this area was limited. It is important to understand what factors explain this result.

The Ministry of Health participated in the nationwide assessment that demonstrated the need to improve access and quality of family planning services (5) and led to the innovations in the Santa Barbara municipality. The project thus followed the basic principle that future "users" of the innovations must be involved from the outset. As time progressed, however, it became more difficult to continue this pattern. In recent years the Ministry has assigned only 4–6 professionals to the national women's health programme, giving them responsibility for obstetric care, gynaecology, adolescent health, early detection of gynaecological cancers and family planning. With this broad range of national responsibilities, the small group of professionals can devote only limited efforts to the improvement of family planning services; consequently it was difficult to maintain their ongoing involvement. Nonetheless, as described below the project sought to engage with state and federal authorities in the three central areas where their intervention could have major impact on scaling up: contraceptive supplies, training resources and financial incentives (25).

Facilitating regular availability of contraceptive supplies

The Brazilian Ministry of Health has declared its commitment to meeting a portion of the municipal need for contraceptive supplies. Municipalities do not have adequate financial resources to provide for their contraceptive needs and the federal government can negotiate better prices with the pharmaceutical industry than can individual municipalities.[5] The Ministry of Health is also in a better position to ensure quality control (7, 37). In previous years, when supplies were available from donors, the Ministry provided contraceptive methods to municipalities if the appropriate requests were made. However, such distribution rarely worked well because municipalities were often unaware of the complex bureaucratic mechanisms involved in submitting their requests.

After the progressive loss of donor contributions in the early 1990s, various efforts were made to distribute contraceptives to municipalities, none of which brought lasting solutions to the supply problem. When the federal government undertook procurement in the mid-1990s, the acquisition of oral contraceptives of unacceptable quality created delays in further action, and subsequently the expectation was that contraceptive procurement would be handled by the states. However, several states refused to include contraceptives in their list of basic medicines, in part because they were afraid quality control problems might be repeated (7). Thereafter, the government planned to provide contraceptive kits to municipalities on a three-month basis, expecting to cover 30% of need in 2001, 60% in 2002, and 100% in 2003. However, the Ministry encountered difficulties with reliable distribu-

---

[5] The need for a continued role of central governments in the provision of contraceptive supplies in decentralized health systems has been noted for other countries as well (16).

tion to the over 5000 municipalities and local storage of supplies. As a result, implementation of the scheme has been irregular (7). In 2004, no kits were distributed for a period of at least six months; subsequently some distribution was resumed.

The Reprolatina Project resource team observed the intricate and evolving variations in federal contraceptive distribution schemes, expecting to assist project municipalities in securing regular supplies once the system was clearly established. The forever changing and unpredictable nature of the process at the federal level, however, left little room for involvement from below. Some of the project municipalities have been able to persuade local authorities to purchase contraceptives. Nonetheless the fact that federal support remains sporadic hinders the process of scaling up family planning innovations.

Mobilizing resources for training

There are few public sector institutions in Brazil that provide in-service training for professionals in family planning and related aspects of reproductive health. The states address the need for human resource development by providing grants to a variety of institutions with relevant training capacity, many of them universities. Scaling up family planning innovations tested by the Reprolatina Project benefited in one region of the country from the availability of such state-level training resources. This became possible because the project was able to establish a close connection to the relevant state-level decision-maker who was convinced of the importance of family planning and has consistently supported logistics and related costs for training programmes organized by the project.

Similar success was not possible in other regions. Because such training funds are not specifically earmarked for family planning but are available for a range of health areas, there is no guarantee that the limited resources can be mobilized for family planning. Success depends on the specific circumstances in each state, especially on the interests of the key decision-maker. Given competing demands on these resources, strong advocacy is required in seeking these funds and many bureaucratic hurdles must be overcome before municipalities succeed.

Lobbying for financial incentives

Influencing financial incentives for family planning was a third area where the Reprolatina Project expected to affect higher-level decision-making in order to institutionalize service innovations pioneered in municipalities. As discussed further in the next section, health sector financing leaves family planning in a position of disadvantage. The project municipalities and the Reprolatina Project resource team discussed the possibilities of influencing the existing pattern of financing with the purpose of ensuring a more favourable incentive structure for family planning.

The suggestion was to bring this issue onto the agenda of the powerful national Council of Municipal Secretaries of Health. However, project municipalities have not been able to accomplish this, in part because of the frequent turnover of health secretaries. More importantly, the project has not pursued this plan because conversations with federal officials indicated that, given the continuing political sensitivities surrounding family planning in Brazil, such proposals would be unlikely to succeed in the near future. The discussion in the next section clarifies these political liabilities.

Thus, overall, the Ministry of Health and the state-level secretariats have not played a strong role in scaling up family planning service innovations originally tested in Santa Barbara. This is so even though these innovations conform to the central agenda of the Brazilian policy framework as most recently articulated in the Family Planning Law (32). As a result, the success with vertical scaling up and institutionalization has been limited.

In theory, the Reprolatina Project resource team could have taken more vigorous advocacy steps with other stakeholders, for example parliamentarians, the National Commission for Population and Development and other national or state-level agencies. The lesson here is that the small NGO resource team had obvious limits in its capacity to advance vertical scaling up. Given the extensive demands for technical assistance and training required in expanding service innovations to new municipalities, a stronger advocacy role of the project at the national and state levels was not feasible.

Political obstacles to scaling up family planning innovations

Considerable progress in the evolution of strong rights-based reproductive health policies has been made in Brazil over the last 15 years. Brazil has shaped the global reproductive health agenda and was itself strongly influenced by international forums such as the 1993 World Conference on Human Rights, Vienna; the 1994 International Conference on Population and Development, Cairo; and the 1995 Fourth World Conference on Women, Beijing. In the past decade, improvements were obtained in hospital-based obstetric services, expansion in prenatal care and cervical cancer screening. New regulations were issued on how the SUS should respond to women who had suffered gender violence, and an increasing number of service sites are providing abortion on grounds permitted by law (38). In 1996 and 1997 the Family Planning Law (32) was enacted, reconfirming family planning as a right within the context of integrated attention to health and obliging the government to provide services respecting each individual's right to choice. A major contribution of this law has been to legalize sterilization, which had been considered semi-illegal, even though it was widely practised. The law also requires that all safe and scientifically proven contraceptive methods are made available.

Although the right of access to contraceptive services is anchored in the Brazilian Constitution, confirmed by the new law and declared important by the Ministry of Health, in practice family planning is not a high priority at either the federal, state or municipal level. No organized set of national or state activities or financial incentives directs the service system to the provision of family planning education and care. At the local level, family planning services are usually among the first to be reduced when municipalities encounter financial constraints or lack of personnel. This position of disadvantage is reflected in health sector financing and can be attributed to the continued religious sensitivities as well as to the overall lack of political appeal of these preventively focused services. As a consequence, efforts to expand family planning innovations are faced with special challenges which would not be encountered in scaling up other reproductive health programmes in Brazil. Understanding how these constraints operate is an essential step in setting realistic scaling-up goals and designing effective strategies.

Family planning's disadvantage in health sector financing

Although health services are controlled at the municipal level, approximately 75% of public sector health-care financing comes from the federal government; the remainder is provided from state and municipal revenues. Federal health financing is provided in the form of per capita allocations, reimbursements for services and financial incentives for special programmes. At the present time, key special programmes supported by the federal government are the safe motherhood and community-based family health initiatives. These are implemented in municipalities that applied for these funds.

Under the SUS each municipality is allocated a fixed per capita amount of about US$ 4 per year. Out of these funds, municipalities should cover primary care including vaccines, maternal health, child nutrition, family planning and tuberculosis treatment (27). In addition to this federal allocation, municipalities are legally committed to devote to health a minimum of 15% annually out of their own budget. Over the past decade, the overall amount of funding for health from federal, state and municipal levels has grown. Because no allocations are designated for contraceptive services, however, family planning competes for funding with other health activities. It rarely does well in this competition, as municipalities are likely to allocate federal funds as well as funds from local revenues for other health priorities, especially curative care.[6] Municipalities often resist requests to purchase contraceptives or purchase them only sporadically, far below actual needs. Previously, when they could request reimbursement from the SUS for services provided, the situation was somewhat better. Although in practice a ceiling was imposed on reimbursements, the system provided an incentive for municipalities to invest in contraceptive services.

Municipalities which have implemented the family health programme can receive additional funds over the Piso de Atençáo Básica (minimum level of services in primary care). Other programmes, such as humanized delivery, also receive special financial incentives. Although such special funds are assigned for primary health care, funds for special programmes cannot be used to purchase contraceptives. Discussion with Ministry representatives revealed that, given the political sensitivities, the prospects for changing the current incentive system in favour of family planning are extremely low.

Religious sensitivities and general lack of political appeal

The political sensitivities surrounding contraception are an important explanation for the low priority accorded to family planning. Even though the Church does not officially oppose family planning, many politicians prefer to support other issues, fearing opposition from local priests who continue to be concerned that methods such as the intrauterine device (IUD) and emergency contraception are abortifacients. For example, in one of the project municipalities, a local law prohibited the use of IUDs, thereby creating a major restriction of contraceptive options available to women. Although this law was in clear violation of federal law, it was passed because of the powerful influence of a local Catholic priest who threatened to shut down the women's health centre if IUDs continued to be provided. After three years of persistent efforts from the women's health coordinator, this law was repealed. The use of IUDs still has not come back to previous levels, in part because the priest continues his campaign against the device.

More recently, religious–political tensions surrounding family planning have coalesced around the issue of emergency contraception, which some local religious groups view as an abortifacient (7). This reaction is so intense that some municipalities are turning entire-

---

[6] The local expenditure choice for curative care has also been observed in other settings. See for example *39*.

ly against family planning, even though federal law clearly approves a broad range of methods including emergency contraception. Decentralization leaves municipalities at liberty to make such decisions because the national government is unable to monitor events at the local level and to enforce federal policies and regulations.

The impact of religious sensitivities is compounded by family planning's lack of political appeal more generally. Mayors seek to maximize their standing with the local electorate and tend to invest in highly visible projects, which demonstrate their contributions in tangible ways. They give priority to building new facilities, buying ambulances, dealing with an epidemic or focusing on child health and see little political advantage in supporting improvements in contraceptive and related reproductive health services. The benefits of family planning and prevention more generally are less obvious to politicians. With the continued high levels of contraceptive prevalence and the increasing availability of Misopristol for medical abortion through the private sector, the argument that family planning saves lives does not carry the same conviction that it did in the past. Equitable access, quality of care and reproductive rights in contraceptive care are not perceived as having the same political pay-offs as other primary health-care initiatives.

Conclusions

Although Brazil's national policy framework is extremely favourable to reproductive health generally and family planning in particular, scaling up family planning service innovations faces extensive constraints. The combination of policy support at the national level and decentralized decision-making can facilitate scaling up, but it can also impede it. The autonomy vested in the municipal governments in the wake of decentralization makes change possible in the many municipalities where interest in these innovations is strong. Such autonomy allows for innovations to be adapted and modified according to local needs. This is a major benefit, because needs vary and particular interventions must be responsive to the local institutional and sociocultural contexts. Inequities arise, however, when there is no interest among municipalities to improve reproductive health services, or when such interest changes over time.[7]

In contrast, the authority to make change also implies that valuable innovations can be swept aside in the face of political change.

---

[7] The fact that decentralization may lead to inequities has been widely discussed in the decentralization literature. See for example *39–41*.

Sustainability at the local level cannot be taken for granted. Over and over again the Reprolatina Project had to shift emphasis from a focus on further expansion to putting energy into sustaining innovations in municipalities where changes in leadership and other personnel threatened continuity. In most cases sustainability could be ensured, but it required extensive support from the project's resource team.

Decentralization provides the context in which political, financial and other institutional factors are played out. In the decentralized, federal setting of Brazil, the Ministry of Health communicates its interest in priority health areas through the mechanism of financial incentives to municipalities. For the political reasons discussed above, contraceptive services have not received such special incentives and are not likely to benefit from them in the near future. Contraceptive services, as well as resources for training, must compete with other pressing primary health-care priorities. Given the continued political sensitivities of family planning and the fact that the benefits of preventive services are not considered as politically rewarding by local decision-makers as are the benefits of curative services, municipalities do not regularly purchase essential contraceptive supplies. The Ministry of Health in turn has sought to provide contraceptive supplies through various schemes but these have not yet succeeded in meeting the need. While federal funds are earmarked for training, they are not necessarily allocated to family planning.

Thus scaling up family planning innovations faces particularly heavy barriers in Brazil. Service innovations related to safe motherhood or the family health programme, for example, would be considerably easier because they benefit from greater priority on the local and national health policy agenda. An important conclusion from this analysis is that the success of scaling up is influenced not only by the intrinsic demands of the service innovations themselves but also by how they fit within the national and local priorities.

What advice can one give to others who seek to ensure successful scaling up in a decentralized setting where successfully tested service innovations do not benefit from high priority on the national and local policy agenda? We list seven key recommendations, which represent the most essential lessons.

1. *Analyse the environmental context of scaling up*. The most general lesson is that understanding the environmental context within which scaling up takes place is vital. Even though a deep understanding of the institutional context for scaling up may at times appear discouraging, it is only when one understands the

system well that the opportunities for positive action become apparent. Examination of the environmental context provides a solid foundation for setting realistic goals and for maximizing existing opportunities.

2. *Focus on sustainability even though this slows down the pace and scope of expansion.* In the long run, fewer but sustainable innovations stand a greater chance of serving as models that can inspire others and generate broader reform than larger expansion that does not survive.

3. *Use national legal and policy frameworks as tools for reproductive health and rights-based training and social mobilization focused on government accountability.* Communities as well as local health authorities and providers are often not well informed about policy and legal advances in reproductive health, nor are they familiar with the mechanisms by which decentralization creates opportunities for resource mobilization. Using such information in training generates demand from below and empowers communities, local authorities and providers to participate effectively in newly created decentralized decision-making forums and advances scaling up.

4. *Use policy windows wisely.* It is essential to keep an eye on policy windows that may open, especially those created by the electoral cycle, and to use the time of such openings wisely. For example, major innovations should not be started at the end of an electoral cycle but at the beginning, so as to maximize the time period in which sustainable innovations can be implemented.

5. *Work with strong municipal teams.* Select municipalities with several strong team members at the level of providers, authorities and the community. This can buffer the effects of frequent change in personnel and ensure sustainability.

6. *Provide training that addresses the rights, gender and reproductive health agenda as well as technical, management and systems needs.* In a decentralized setting where more responsibility for programme design and management falls upon local health teams than in a centralized setting, sustainable scaling up requires training that prepares health teams and communities for a broader range of competencies than was needed in the past. Training should generate a vision of what is possible within the constrained context, create commitment to achieving it, address the need for effective technical and managerial skills, and empower the team to move forward together.

7. *Ensure the availability of an external resource team with long time horizons and the ability to support both vertical and horizontal scaling up.* Continuity from an external resource team over a number of years ensures sustainability of the scaling-up process because longer time horizons make it possible to outlast short-term political change.

The analysis in this chapter reinforces the wisdom that scaling up should be based on an understanding of the context or environment within which it takes place. Such analysis should be ongoing because the institutional context does not stay frozen in time. This is particularly true as long as decentralization is still in the process of being shaped and finalized. Such change may provide new opportunities, but it may also imply that old solutions do not work any longer and new ones need to be discovered. In decentralized and constrained political settings, scaling up must begin with the willingness to engage in a learning process.

Acknowledgments

This paper has benefited greatly from the many reviews by our colleagues; we especially wish to thank Peter Fajans, Laura Ghiron, Max Heirich and Jeremy Shiffman for their valuable inputs. We are extremely grateful for the financial support we received from the Bill and Melinda Gates Foundation, the Rockefeller Foundation and the University of Michigan.

References

1. Paul S. *Managing development programs: the lessons of success.* Boulder, CO, Westview Press, 1982.

2. *Pesquisa Nacional por Amostra de Domicilios (PNAD) 2003, Utilização de servicos de saúde [Demographic and Health Survey 2003, Utilization of health services].* Instituto Brasileiro de Geografia e Estatística (IBGE), 2003 (http://www.ibge.gov.br/home/estatistica/populacao/trabalhoerendimento/pnad2003/saude/comentario.pdf, accessed 5 April 2006).

3. *O desenvolvimento do Sistema Único de Saúde: avanços, desafios e reafirmação dos seus princípios e diretrizes. [The development of the unified system of health: advances, challenges and reaffirmation of its principles and guidelines].* Brasília, DF, Ministério da Saúde, Conselho Nacional de Saúde, 2002 (Série B, Textos básicos de Saúde [Series B, Basic Texts on Health]).

4. Member Association: Brazil. New York, International Planned Parenthood Federation (http:www.ippfwhr.org/profiles/association_e.asp?AssociationID=3, accessed 17 February 2006).

5. Formiga JN, Simmons R, Cravey E et al. *An assessment of the need for contraceptive introduction in Brazil*. Geneva, World Health Organization, 1994 (Special Programme of Research, Development and Research Training in Human Reproduction, WHO/HRP/ITT/94.2).

6. Giffin K. Women's health and the privatization of fertility control in Brazil. *Social Science and Medicine*, 1994, 39:355–360.

7. *Relatório: Seminário política de anticoncepção no Sistema Único de Saúde (SUS) [Report: Seminar on contraceptive policies within the Unified Health System]*. Brasília, DF, Ministério da Saúde, Conselho Nacional de Saúde & Comissão Intersectorial de Saúde da Muhler, 2001 (http://conselho.saude.gov.br/comissao/docs/SEMIN%C1RIO%20POL%CDTICA%20DE%20ANTICONCEP%C7%C3O%20NO%20SUS.rtf, accessed 17 February 2006).

8. Díaz M, Simmons R. When is research participatory? Reflections on a reproductive health project in Brazil. *Journal of Women's Health*, 1999, 8:175–184.

9. Penteado LG, Cabral F, Díaz M et al. Organizing a public sector vasectomy program in Brazil. *Studies in Family Planning*, 2001, 32:315–328.

10. Díaz M, Simmons R, Díaz J et al. Expanding contraceptive choice: findings from Brazil. *Studies in Family Planning*, 1999, 30:1–16.

11. Simmons R, Hall P, Díaz J et al. The strategic approach to contraceptive introduction. *Studies in Family Planning*, 1997, 28:79–94.

12. *The strategic approach to improving reproductive health policies and programmes: a summary of experiences*. Geneva, World Health Organization, 2002 (Department of Reproductive Health and Research, WHO/RHR/02.12).

13. Fajans P, Simmons R, Ghiron L. Helping public-sector health systems innovate: the strategic approach for strengthening reproductive health policies and programs. *American Journal of Public Health*, 2006, 96:2–7.

14. Simmons R, Brown JW, Díaz M. Facilitating large-scale transitions to quality of care. *Studies in Family Planning*, 2002, 33:61–75.

15. *Evaluating World Health Organization Project 96323: Brazil Stage III: Researching the utilization and dissemination of findings from a project on the improvement of contraceptive choice within the context of reproductive health. Final technical report*. São Paulo, Centro de Pesquisas Materno-Infantis de Campinas (CEMICAMP) [Centre for Mother and Child Research of Campinas], 2000 (unpublished).

16. Aitken IW. Implications of decentralization as a reform strategy for the implementation of reproductive health programs. In: *The implications of health sector reform for reproductive health and rights*. Washington, DC, CHANGE/Population Council, 1998 (Report of a meeting of the Working Group for Reproductive Health and Family Planning).

17. Langer A, Nigenda G, Catino J. Health sector reform and reproductive health in Latin America and the Caribbean: strengthening the links. *Bulletin of the World Health Organization*, 2000, 78:667–676.

18. World Health Organization. Health sector reform – the implications for reproductive health services. *Progress in Reproductive Health Research*, 2005, 69:1–8.

19. Atkinson S, Medeiros RLR, Oliveira PHL et al. Going down to the local: incorporating social organization and political culture into assessments of decentralized health care. *Social Science and Medicine*, 2000, 51:619–636.

20. Weyland K. Social movements and the state: the politics of health reform in Brazil. *World Development*, 1995, 23:1699–1712.

21. Collins C, Araujo J, Barbosa J. Decentralizing the health sector: issues in Brazil. *Health Policy*, 2000, 52:113–127.

22. Lobato L. Reorganizing the health care system in Brazil. In: Fleury S, Belmartino S, Baris E, eds. *Reshaping health care in Latin America: a comparative analysis of health care reform in Argentina, Brazil and Mexico*. Geneva, International Development Research Centre, 2000:103–132.

23. Elias P, Cohn A. Health reform in Brazil: lessons to consider. *American Journal of Public Health*, 2003, 93:44–48.

24. *Coleção Políticas prioritárias do Instituto Nacional de Assistência Médica da Previdência Social (INAMPS) (1985–1988) [Collection of priority policies of the National Institute of Medical Care of the Social Welfare System (1985–1988)]*. Rio de Janeiro, FIOCRUZ, 2005 (http://www.coc.fiocruz.br/areas/dad/guia_acervo/arq_pessoal/colecao_inamps.htm, accessed 17 February 2006).

25. Sistema Único de Saúde (SUS). Aspectos gerais [Unified Health System. General aspects] (http://www.sespa.pa.gov.br/SUS/sus/sus_aspgerais.htm, accessed 17 February 2006).

26. *Norma Operacional Básica do Sistema Único de Saúde – SUS/NOB-SUS 96 [Basic operational norm of the Unified Health System]*. Brasília, Ministério da Saúde, Diário Oficial da União, 6 November 1996.

27. *Regionalização da assistência à saúde: aprofundando a descentralização com eqüidade no acesso, norma operacional da assistência à saúde [Regionalization of health care: strengthening decentralization with equitable access, operational norms of health care].* Brasília, DF, Ministério da Saúde, Secretaria de Assistência à Saúde, 2001:114 (NOAS-SUS 01/01, e Portaria MS/GM n. 95, de 26 de janeiro de 2001, e regulamentação complementar. Série A, Normas e manuais técnicos [Series A, Norms and Technical Manuals], No. 116).

28. *SUS – 15 anos de implantação. Desafios e propostas para sua consolidação [SUS – 15 years of implementation. Challenges and proposals for its consolidation].* Brasília, DF, Ministério da Saúde, 2003 (Série Políticas de Saúde [Series Politics and Health]).

29. Número de municípios habilitados – situação junho 2005 [Number of qualified municipalities – situation as of June 2005]. Brasilia, Ministério da Saúde, 2005 (http://dtr2001.saude.gov.br/dad, accessed 18 February, 2006).

30. *Going to scale: can we bring more benefits to more people more quickly?* Silang, Cavite, Philippines, International Institute of Rural Reconstruction, Y.C. James Yen Center, 2000.

31. Guendel S, Jancock J, Anderson S. *Scaling-up strategies for research in natural resources management: a comparative review.* Chatham, Natural Resources Institute, 2001.

32. Lei N. 9263 de 12 de janeiro de 1996 [Law No 9236, 12 January 1996]. Brasília, Ministério da Saúde, Diário Oficial da União, 15 January 1996.

33. *Planajamento Familiar. Manual para o gestor [Family planning. Manual for the manager].* Brasília, DF, Ministério da Saúde, 2002 (Série A, Normas e manuais técnicos [Series A, Norms and Technical Manuals]).

34. *Assistência em planejamento familiar. Manual técnico [Assistance in family planning services. Technical manual],* 4th ed. Brasília, DF, Ministério da Saúde, 2002 (Série A, Normas e manuais técnicos [Series A, Norms and Technical Manuals], No. 40).

35. Haines A. Health care in Brazil. *British Medical Journal,* 1993, 306:503–512.

36. Presidência da República. *Mensagem Nº 928, de 19 de agosto de 1997 [Decree Number 928, 19 August 1997].* Brasília, DF, Diário Oficial da União, 1997.

37. Araújo MJ, Melo J. Saúde da mulher é prioridade no ministério – entrevistas com Tania Lago [Women's health is priority in the ministry – interviews with Tania Lago]. *Jornal da Rede Feminista de Saúde*, 2000, No. 20 (http://www.redesaude.org.br/jornal/html/jr20-tania.html, accessed 17 February 2006).

38. Corrêa S, McIntyre P, Rodrigues C et al. The population and reproductive health programme in Brazil 1990–2002: lessons learned. *Reproductive Health Matters*, 2005, 13:72–80.

39. Bossert TJ, Beauvais JC. Decentralization of health systems in Ghana, Zambia, Uganda and the Philippines: a comparative analysis of decision space. *Health Policy and Planning*, 2002, 17:14–31.

40. Collins C, Green A. Decentralization and primary health care: some negative implications in developing countries. *International Journal of Health Services*, 1994, 24:459–475.

41. Isaacs S, Solimano G. Health reform and civil society in Latin America. *Development*, 1999, 42:70–72.

Chapter 8

An innovative educational approach to capacity building and scaling up reproductive health services in Latin America

Margarita Díaz, Francisco Cabral[a]

Summary

As governments seek to meet the global health agendas of the past decade, new approaches to the training of health professionals are needed. Training must move away from an exclusive focus on technical skills and begin to incorporate educational strategies that empower providers, programme managers and community leaders to become agents of change. This chapter describes a methodology for in-service training that builds on Paulo Freire's educational philosophy and explains how the capacity to provide innovative training was scaled up in public sector reproductive health services in Brazil, Bolivia and Chile. Statistics on the training sessions demonstrate the reach of this training initiative, and testimonials show its profound impact on newly trained trainers.

Introduction

The 1994 International Conference on Population and Development (ICPD), held in Cairo, as well as several subsequent international summits, challenged governments to implement far-reaching goals in reproductive and primary health care, gender and women's empowerment, and the eradication of poverty and major diseases (1–3). At the same time, many national governments have been striving to enact changes in their health systems in the wake of decentralization and health sector reform. Realizing the vision of these global and national agendas requires a process of social transformation that includes changes in the attitudes of health authorities, managers, providers and the community. In this chapter we argue that working towards

---

[a] Margarita Díaz is President and Francisco Cabral is Vice-president of Reprolatina; they designed and implemented the training methodology described in this paper.

such changes has major implications for training, because training is one of the main tools by which new attitudes and skills can be developed.

Given the magnitude of change implied in the necessary transformation, training itself has to change. It must move away from an exclusive focus on technical skills and from biological notions of reproductive health that give little consideration to social, cultural and political dimensions. Training must incorporate educational strategies that will allow providers, programme managers and community leaders to become agents of change. Without such empowerment, the massive reform implied in global visions cannot be achieved. The challenge is to develop innovative approaches and to build the capacity for widespread utilization and scaling up of new and empowering training methodologies in public sector service systems.

We had the opportunity to develop such a new approach and to demonstrate how the capacity to provide innovative in-service training could be expanded within the public sector. This chapter describes the key elements of the training methodology and shows how it was developed in one municipality in Brazil and was subsequently scaled up to several others and extended to Bolivia and Chile. This chapter identifies how a small nongovernmental team can initiate change and build public sector training capacity that orients managers, providers and community leaders to new visions of reproductive health.

The information presented here is based on four sources of data: our own experience as sexual and reproductive health trainers; focus groups with newly trained trainers, which we conducted in July–November 2005 with six groups in Brazil and one each in Bolivia and Chile; in-depth interviews we conducted with municipal health and local government authorities in July–November 2005 (11 in Brazil, 2 in Bolivia, and 9 in Chile); and project statistics on the number of training programmes conducted.

Evolution of Reprolatina's training approach

The opportunity to develop innovative training presented itself first in connection with the implementation of the Strategic Approach to Strengthening Reproductive Health Policies and Programmes sponsored by the World Health Organization (WHO) (4, 5) and subsequently with the Reprolatina Project, an initiative funded by the Bill and Melinda Gates Foundation. Strategic assessments, undertaken first in Brazil (1993) and subsequently in Bolivia (1995) and Chile (1996), revealed glaring shortcomings in the provision of public sector reproductive health services (6, 7). Although there were differences among the findings in the three countries, the assessments identified similar weaknesses. Access to reproductive health care and to quality family planning services was extremely constrained, and health-care providers' technical knowledge was outdated. Interpersonal relations reflected the power, class and ethnic differentials between providers and local people and were not conducive to interactions that educate or empower the participants. The sexual and reproductive health and rights vision articulated in Cairo was not present in day-to-day health-care delivery, and providers and managers were not prepared to incorporate its multiple challenges into their work.

In 1995 the Center for Mother and Child Research of Campinas (CEMICAMP) initiated an action research project to test appropriate responses to the assessment findings in a low-income municipality. The Population Council and the University of Michigan collaborated with this project and financial support was provided by WHO (8, 9). Focus on a municipality was dictated by the fact that in the decentralized setting of Brazil programmatic decisions about service delivery are made at the municipal level (see Chapter 7). The Santa Barbara Project – named after the municipality in which it was implemented – used a participatory organization development approach, in which municipal providers, health authorities, community representatives and researchers worked in close collaboration.[1] They began with a diagnostic assessment to establish specific needs; followed by designing and implementing interventions, and ongoing evaluation. The main interventions focused on:

- upgrading all elements of quality of care (11);
- restructuring providers' roles and service delivery patterns so as to maximize the use of scarce medical personnel;
- improving the management process in order to ensure accountability and supportive supervision;
- creating a referral centre where contraceptive services would be available on a regular basis;
- establishing a participatory process of project decision-making with representation from the community (12);
- introducing outpatient vasectomy services (13);

---

[1] Organization development is defined as "a long-term effort, led and supported by top management, to improve an organization's visioning, empowerment, learning and problem-solving processes, through an ongoing, collaborative management of organization culture ... utilizing the consultant-facilitator role and the theory and technology of applied behavioural science, including action research" (10, p. 28).

- developing a programme for adolescents.

As described later, these interventions were supported with training programmes for all members of the municipal health team.

Evaluation results in 1997 indicated that these interventions substantially improved both quality and access to family planning and related reproductive health care in the municipality (8). At this stage the project began to turn its attention to scaling up, asking whether expansion of the successful interventions to other municipalities in Brazil would be feasible. Initial scaling up was undertaken in three municipalities with support from WHO and proved successful (14). This led to further expansion within Brazil and the initiation of activities in Bolivia and Chile between 1999 and 2006 through the Reprolatina Project, which created training capacity in nine municipalities in Brazil, eight in Bolivia and three in Chile (for the sake of simplicity we use the term "municipality" for Bolivia and Chile, though other terms are used locally).

Training was provided by a resource team consisting of ourselves and colleagues, first from CEMICAMP and subsequently from Reprolatina, a small Brazilian nongovernmental organization (NGO) created in 1999. This training was instrumental in producing the project's success and, as we describe below, was a key component of the scaling-up strategy. One of us (M.D.) had had many years of experience in training family planning providers in Brazil and other countries of Latin America and had already begun to recognize that training on technical aspects of contraceptive care needed to be complemented with a focus on interpersonal relations, gender and sexuality. In the course of implementing the training first in Santa Barbara and in the subsequent scaling up in Brazil, Bolivia and Chile, this perspective evolved further.

Such evolution occurred along two dimensions. First, it quickly became apparent that training topics needed to be broadened to take account of the multiple needs and problems faced by the municipal health teams. For example, teams were not used to identifying their own problems and finding solutions within their resource constraints. Training thus had to be holistic, seeking to build and sustain capacity through a comprehensive educational approach that enables local teams to analyse their own reality and empowers them to change it, and to provide good sexual and reproductive health care. Second, it was clear that Reprolatina trainers had to develop the capacity of the municipal team to assume training tasks – so that they could train others within the municipality and expand training to neighbouring municipalities. With this recognition, the strategy of the resource team shifted from training of providers to training of trainers in a broad, empowerment-focused educational approach.[2]

Reprolatina's educational philosophy

Reprolatina's educational philosophy builds on Paulo Freire's understanding that thinking critically about current and past practices allows us to improve the world in which we live (15–17). Freire argued that people can act as oppressors or as liberators of their own situation, and emphasized that the purpose of education is to create autonomous persons who engage with a project of emancipation. The objective of such an educational process is to transform current social structures (18).

Reprolatina considers education and health to be closely interrelated. The philosophy emphasizes that individuals have unique personal histories and live within a social, political, economic and cultural environment that influences them but that they also shape. Each person has unique knowledge, including those who never attended school. All people have the right and capacity to think, take part in dialogue, have opinions and make choices.

Typically, however, the education and health sectors do not give people the opportunity to participate in decisions about their lives. Education systems are built on power imbalances and passive approaches to learning. This model is repeated in the health profession, which typically treats people as patients or objects of programmes rather than as agents of transformation who participate in their own health care. To put the Cairo agenda into practice, the educational process in the health and the education sectors must change – promoting social and gender equality and encouraging the development of citizens with rights and responsibilities.

Reprolatina begins work in a new municipality by introducing an innovative educational process which, in turn, generates new ways of managing and providing services in reproductive health and facilitates scaling up. At the outset, the Reprolatina team takes the lead in the educational process, acting both as teacher and learner. Working in a participatory way, the team at times transfers new ideas; on other occasions, the team receives new ideas from the participants.

Reprolatina's educational strategy has four interrelated goals. The first, which is the essential precondition for the other three, focuses on

[2] Key dimensions of empowerment as used in Reprolatina's training programme include the ability to take decisions about one's life, effective expression of one's human rights as well as physical and emotional needs, capability to reflect collectively about one's experiences, and the ability to organize and articulate one's demands at local, national and international levels vis-à-vis governments and other institutions.

personal and professional empowerment. In order to be empowered, health providers must go through a process of reflection and self-evaluation to be able to identify why they should change. Before health professionals can provide a new standard of care they must discover their own ability to introduce changes that will improve the quality of care they provide. Training aims to enable individuals to be active participants in the learning process and to become dedicated agents of change. It takes into account the life experience, knowledge, expectations and self-esteem of learners and addresses cognitive, cultural and affective aspects including the feelings that emerge during the training process. Participants are expected to develop a greater sense of self-awareness and autonomy as well as a common sense of solidarity.

The second dimension addresses *knowledge and technical skills*. Training provides accurate technical information that is offered at a level appropriate to the knowledge of different participants. Areas covered include knowledge and awareness of the human body, sexuality, power, and sexual and gender roles, as well as practical training on contraception and related aspects of reproductive health care. Training also develops counselling and communication skills to help participants improve communications within the health team and to interact supportively with service users.

A third dimension of training deals with the need to create the capacity for *organization development* so that trainees will be able to promote changes in the health system. Trainees are sensitized to the importance of understanding the characteristics of the health system that create and sustain current problems in quality of care and of the social and economic characteristics of the community they serve. Participants acquire the ability to diagnose problems, to identify opportunities for intervention and to test their proposed solutions and evaluate them. Simultaneously, they develop negotiation skills and learn how to work more effectively as a team and to undertake self-evaluation. Participants learn about and acquire the needed skills to conduct supervision and empowerment-focused evaluation (*19*).

The fourth goal of training is developing the capacity to act as facilitator for *social and cultural transformation*. Participants develop critical understanding of the social, economic and cultural dynamics that shape current health policies and practices, and the power relations that govern these dynamics, including tensions between the public and private health sectors. They gain a clearer understanding of the meaning and role that gender and power play in their health system and in people's lives. Participants are trained to become trainers and facilitators of a process of change.

The process of capacity building

Building capacity to improve health service systems is a complex undertaking. It requires appropriate training programmes as well as efforts to create an enabling environment where training can succeed. These are not short-term interventions but initiatives requiring considerable investment of time and energy.

Types of training programmes

Reprolatina has assembled a range of training courses for health providers, educators, adolescents and community leaders.

Reprolatina's most important curriculum is for the training of trainers, which is provided by a midwife (M.D.) and a psychologist (F.C.) with the support of a physician from the Population Council, Brazil, who provides training on the technical aspects of contraceptive methods. Reprolatina begins by carefully selecting a group of up to 20 participants from among the team of municipal health providers (physicians, nurses, midwives, psychologists and social workers). Selection is based on the candidates' potential and previous experience as trainers, their past work in family planning and reproductive health, their commitment to complete the 80-hour course, and their ability to devote enough time to conduct at least one training course every other month. These conditions often limit the number of providers who qualify, but this selection process helps to ensure that the most appropriate providers receive the training.

The training-of-trainers curriculum is taught in two stages, each consisting of a 40-hour course. The first course begins with basic principles, concepts and values such as sexual and reproductive health and rights, gender, quality of care, informed choice and the user perspective. Subsequently the course moves to the development of skills and competencies focused on client-centred interpersonal relations, communication, counselling and provision of contraceptive methods. Skills development also covers participatory approaches, organization development and health systems analysis. In addition, the course includes attention to special topics such as adolescent sexual and reproductive health, sexuality, and HIV/AIDS. Trainees also learn about the experience of the Santa Barbara Project and the objective of scaling up pilot interventions more broadly in the country.

Between the first and second course is a break of approximately two months so that trainees can read the literature they are given upon completion of the first training. This literature includes publications on the Strategic Approach, the Santa Barbara Project, scaling up, organization development, informed choice, reproductive rights, gender and Freire's educational philosophy. During this break, trainees also conduct a baseline diagnosis in their municipalities to assess community perspectives and needs in sexual and reproductive health as well as service access and quality at the primary care level in the public sector. Reprolatina provides training in how to conduct such a baseline diagnosis as well as instruments for interviewing members of the local community and local clinic staff, and for conducting observations of service provision and facilities. This diagnosis provides the basis for action planning subsequent to the completion of the training-of-trainers programme.

The second course prepares trainees for their role as trainers and leaders who will improve quality and access to sexual and reproductive health services in their municipality. It treats the issues covered in the basic training in greater depth, analysing in detail Reprolatina's philosophy and conceptual frameworks and providing specific training in educational methods, learning processes and group management. With this training behind them, the newly trained trainers are ready to replicate the basic training course (the same they received in the first 40-hour course) using the manual prepared for this purpose.[3]

In family planning, newly trained trainers offer either a 40-hour course or a shorter 24-hour course covering the same topics but in less detail. It is preferred that every member of the municipal health team receives the longer training, but the shorter course is given when either the trainer or the trainees do not have sufficient time for the longer one.

A team approach is used in training so that doctors, nurses, receptionists, social workers and psychologists are trained together. Such team training is essential to create an egalitarian environment where everyone's role receives respect and teamwork is practised. The first course conducted by new trainers is supervised by a member of the Reprolatina team who facilitated their training. Most of the trainers are able to continue on their own after this first observed training. They have a goal to train at least 80% of the providers in their municipality. Funding for such training is provided by the municipality, while Reprolatina provides the training materials.

In addition to the training-of-trainers curriculum, Reprolatina has developed several other courses related to its adolescent programme, community participation, sexually transmitted infections (STIs) and HIV/AIDS, sexuality, breastfeeding, and screening for breast and cervical cancer. Reprolatina also organizes shorter seminars for physi-

---

[3] The manual includes detailed instructions on how to manage each module, the time allocated for each activity and the summary points. An annex contains guidelines for participatory techniques, a bibliography, and a CD-ROM with all the slides to be used during training.

cians and other professionals who are not able to attend regular-length training courses. These 8-hour seminars cover the philosophy of rights, gender and quality of care – though obviously more briefly than the other training programmes – and update provider knowledge of contraceptive technology and prevention and treatment of STIs. In some cases Reprolatina also provides additional practical training on insertion of intrauterine devices (IUDs), Pap smear collection, how to fit diaphragms, and how to do non-scalpel vasectomy.

All of Reprolatina's training curricula are available to trainers who wish to use them in their municipality. For some of the courses, Reprolatina is able to provide additional training, for others it provides materials and slides that update providers on subjects with which they are already familiar.

In addition to their role as trainers, participants who have completed both courses are expected to act as a leadership team that will work with other providers to improve services in their municipality. During the training they had opportunity to learn from the innovations that succeeded in Santa Barbara and other municipalities in Brazil. The results from the diagnostic assessment they conducted between the two training courses provide the basis for determining which of the pilot innovations should be scaled up in their municipality and what other interventions should be undertaken.

The first activity the trainers are supposed to implement is establishing a training centre. They identify a place to meet at least once a month and to keep their computing equipment and other materials. Such a meeting place is essential because trainers work in different health centres within the municipality and they need a meeting place where they can plan training as well as other initiatives. Thereafter they begin the process of conducting training courses for providers as well as implementing necessary changes in service delivery identified during the baseline diagnosis undertaken in their municipality.

Creating an enabling environment for training

Training programmes often fail to have lasting impact. Recognizing from the outset that capacity building is not a short or easy process, Reprolatina seeks to create an enabling environment in each new municipality which ensures that the training-of-trainers programme and other innovations can be successfully introduced, sustained and expanded. Three measures are essential in this process: political commitment and participation of the municipal government and local health authorities; empowerment-focused supervision; and an electronic information system to facilitate communication among participating municipalities and Reprolatina.

Political commitment and participation. Reprolatina signs an agreement with the state and/or municipal health authorities in the regions in the three countries where activities are being implemented. In these agreements the government endorses the creation of training capacity in the municipality, authorizes the participation of providers in the training programme and its subsequent replication and promises necessary support. Such formalized agreements between Reprolatina and each municipality have been instrumental in sustaining activities when local governments changed in the wake of elections.

Political commitment has been instrumental in maintaining activities when resources are scarce. On several occasions, municipal authorities have provided extra resources for new staff, information, education and communication (IEC) materials, contraceptive methods and other unforeseen needs. Nonetheless, regular municipal financing for these activities is not guaranteed.

Empowerment-focused evaluation and coaching. Capacity building requires performance evaluation that reinforces newly trained trainers in their role as innovators. In providing such support, Reprolatina staff work with the principles of empowerment evaluation, which is "designed to help people help themselves and improve their programmes using a form of self-evaluation and reflection" (*20*, p. 3). Trainers are taught to evaluate their activities and use results to plan new ones. These constitute entirely new approaches for most trainees, who are used to a narrow approach to supervision which is focused on administrative compliance. Similarly, when Reprolatina staff observe service delivery, they act as coaches rather than as conventional supervisors. The emphasis is not on criticism but on encouragement of self-evaluation, sharing of experience and reflection.

Electronic communication. When the volume of communication between Reprolatina and municipalities and among municipalities increased rapidly early in the project, an appropriate system was needed to manage it. A communication network was built, using WebBoard™ and three web sites, with technical support from the School of Information at the University of Michigan. This has proven to be efficient. All the trained personnel having an e-mail address were invited to participate in this electronic network and they all received information, bulletins and IEC materials through the network. To date, 71% of trained personnel have access to a computer. The three web sites provide updated technical information and project information to project partners and the community at large. One of the sites describes the philosophy, history and activities of the Reprolatina Project (http://www.reprolatina.net); the second, entitled Living Adolescence, provides correct and up-to-date information for adolescents on diverse subjects of sexual and reproductive health and rights (http://www.adolescencia.org.br); and the third, Contraception Online, is an extensive online resource for sexual and reproductive health information related to technical aspects of contraception (http://www.anticoncepcao.org.br).

Results

Scaling up training capacity

The first training of trainers was performed in 2000 in Brazil, in 2001 in Bolivia and in 2002 in Chile. Table 8.1 shows the number of training centres created and the number of trainers and providers trained per country, including providers attending 8-hour seminars for updating knowledge on family planning and STIs. An important indicator of training capacity is the fact that providers were trained by the newly trained trainers. The table, however, hides the variability of the results. Although the capacity-building process was implemented similarly in all sites, some centres were able to begin replication of the activities soon after training and needed only short-term supervisory support, while other centres were not able to expand the process.

Figure 8.1 shows the multiplicative scaling-up process in Brazil, in which Reprolatina-trained trainers are scaling up the process to other municipalities. The Ministry of Health and state governments have also been participants in this process, mainly by giving political support and financial resources in some cases.

	Number of training centres/ teams	Number of trainers trained	Number of providers trained	Number of providers attending 8-hour seminars
Brazil (2000–2005)	9	98	1921	1219
Bolivia (2001–2005)	8	34	741	758
Chile (2002–2005)	3	21	395	47
Total	**20**	**153**	**3057**	**2024**

Table 8.1 Training outputs

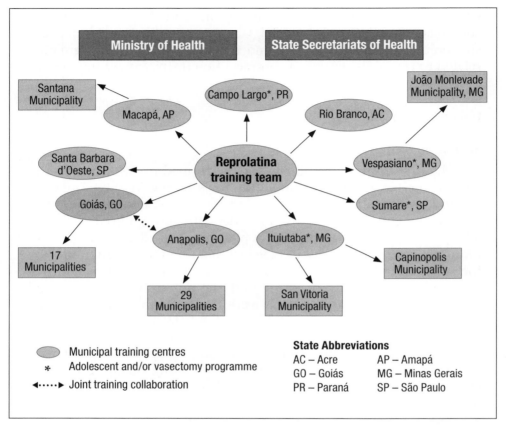

Figure 8.1 Scaling up training capacity in Brazilian municipalities

Building training capacity has progressed at different speeds in different places, because of political and administrative issues that either interfered with or facilitated the process (see Chapter 7). In some places, additional resources were mobilized. For example, in the State of Goiás the project was expanded to 38 municipalities with partial financing from the state level; another municipality in the State of Minas Gerais started scaling up with financial support from a private national foundation, Fundação Belgo. In Bolivia it was possible to expand the training capacity to four additional teams with the support of the United Nations Population Fund (UNFPA).

Most municipalities focused on scaling up innovations that improved existing reproductive health services. In some communities, however, scaling up also added new services for men or adolescents which previously had not been available, but had been tested in Santa Barbara. This required additional training, especially for the adolescent programme.

Trainers' testimonials

Perception of training impact and methodology. The Reprolatina training programme left a deep impression on participants.[4] It challenged them to reflect on their professional work and their personal goals. Concepts such as sexual and reproductive health, informed choice and reproductive rights are not just new technical terms for them but ideas that have transformed the way they look at their work and relate to others. Trainees feel connected – some of them for the first time – to the basic values of their profession, and talk about the new perspectives with which they look at service users, community members and also their colleagues. Extracts from some of their comments are given below, with the municipality and country of the respondent indicated in parentheses.

> *It's as if you light a candle in a person so that she knows she has a mission and is not alone; she has someone who stands behind all of this and gives support so that she is in a position to change.* (Macapá, Brazil)

> *I had never seen anything like this. I can say with complete certainty that this totally changed my way of looking at health, of looking at the world.* (Campo Largo, Brazil)

> *If I could put it in one word, this word would be "transformation", because… you enter in the process as one person and then it seems that this person flourishes, as pop-corn that explodes in knowledge and willingness of doing and modifying things, and begin having a different vision, not that technical but a very humanized vision … a stimulus so great that you feel willing and excited and wanting to work.* (Anápolis, Brazil)

> *The approach you gave on how to treat the users, the integrated care, this I liked very much, really it motivated me. One was used to talking about contraceptive methods and wanting to impose them. In Reprolatina the exercise of the right, that the person looks what is more convenient and one only orients her to what she can or cannot use, using the eligibility criteria … That was the most important: the approach and our change of the attitude.* (Santa Cruz, Bolivia)

---

[4] The evidence presented in this section is based on focus group discussions (using standard focus group methodology) and in-depth interviews conducted with trained trainers in 2005 in Brazil, Bolivia and Chile, as part of the participatory and formative evaluation component of Reprolatina's training programme. Given that the interviewers were also the trainers there is likely to be a courtesy bias in these comments. Nonetheless, it is revealing to hear the words of the trainees describing how the training affected them.

No other training has this empowerment so that people come out from here with a sense of responsibility, knowing what they can do, that they can transform; that it is a process of transformation which is complicated and difficult and lengthy, ... that's what I learned from you. ... Much needs to be changed here, but you opened this space for people. (Macapá, Brazil)

I had at times difficulty to relate to my place of work and to the people ... I was stubborn and not tolerant ... I saw that I changed ... I now consider myself a better professional, I am better prepared, more attentive, not only in terms of knowledge but as a person, as a human being, and I can see that I can contribute more as a colleague. (Ituiutaba, Brazil)

One of the things that affected me most was the part on sexuality, which led me to reflect; this is a part that has a different perspective. The other thing that also affected me ... was the gender focus ... .And for sure, the case of Paulo Freire – this methodology affected me. (Temuco, Chile)

I will always be grateful to you for the flipchart. I take it wherever I go ... Once when there were 35 women gathered together ... to hear about contraceptive methods, a woman said to me she had never heard an explanation about methods like this. And I felt fulfilled because I never had imagined that I would be able to communicate in this way. (Campo Largo, Brazil)

In no other workshops I attended did it happen that at the end of the 40 hours I had the same enthusiasm as when I was in the workshop. The different approach on how to treat the users, how to treat ourselves, to discover that we were closed, blind ... for me it was like awaking to another world and another vision regarding choice, consent. (Santa Cruz, Bolivia)

The profoundly challenging and provocative nature of the training was expressed in the statement that sometimes the training was so intense and covered so many important issues that at times it made people

think too much ... and at times robbed them of their sleep. In some moments I did not like some of the discussions but today I see that these were necessary. (Ituiutaba, Brazil)

The training methodology used by the Reprolatina team was different from that which most participants had experienced in previous training courses, and was viewed as effective and inspiring. For example, the leader of a woman's health centre commented that seeing democratic leadership during the training affirmed her own leadership style. She realized that her own style was not wrong, and that it was good to be flexible, open and friendly with team members (Itu-iutaba, Brazil). Others had similar views:

> *What I noted in the second training was the manner in which you sold the fish (that is) the methodology which you used. There was no way we could get out of there without incorporating Reprolatina's style, and beyond the knowledge, of course, the manner in which you approached the subject. Sometimes you were in the skin of the patient, then you acted as the professional, this was very interesting.* (Campo Largo, Brazil)

> *I liked the participation, the exchange of information, each speaking from his or her own experience, the opportunity we had to speak, to discuss. This really was very different from all the courses I had previously.* (Macapá, Brazil)

> *I found the methodology interesting ... people absorb it, assimilate it. And this was incorporated in what people do. It's not a separate thing that is imposed by you, but one assimilates it in a natural way and there is a natural incorporation into one's work.* (Rio Branco, Brazil)

Replicating the training. Training municipal providers, using Reprolatina's methodology, was initially not easy for most newly trained trainers. They were nervous, uncertain whether they would succeed, and in some cases encountered initial resistance from the participants of the course they organized. However, most found that their initial anxiety disappeared and that they were capable of overcoming difficulties and succeeded in providing a good course. All agreed that in addition to the methodology, the training manual, the slides and all the materials were crucial for the success of replication.

> *The first day I was ready to die, you don't know how the group will be, you don't know whether there will be people who will ask many questions, you don't know whether they will all keep their mouths shut, and what you will do so that they will talk – this is the dilemma until you get to know the group ... The second or third day is much easier, ... when you reach the fourth day you wish it would continue and when you reach the last day you realize that everything has been accomplished, that you succeeded and that is very good.* (Campo Largo, Brazil)

> *I was extremely stressed before my first training. I studied a lot; it seemed as if I was going take an exam ... But when the time arrived it was a delight. It was so good, everything was fluent ... I did not feel afraid at that moment. In the beginning I was insecure, with much fear,*

also because of my own lack of study, because one needs to prepare a lot in order to be in front of people. Even then, people saw the results … the unity of the group, the commitment of the group … it was very good. (Ituiutaba, Brazil)

Success with improving service delivery and sexual and reproductive rights. The Reprolatina resource team observed important changes after the training that improved sexual and reproductive rights and health services in project municipalities. These included obtaining a new building for a health centre, persuading municipal authorities to purchase contraceptives, improving patient flow and the way the service staff related to clients, maintaining patient registers, increasing the volume of contraceptive services, expanding the type of methods used, implementing the informed choice process, and providing participatory educational activities and counselling sessions. Trainees also commented on these changes:

I have helped disseminate sexual rights and not only in the area of health but also in other instances in the community. Moreover, the whole team has done this as well. (Temuco, Chile)

In terms of physical infrastructure people battled and requested Dr X … to make a visit so that he could see the reality of our women's centre, how precarious it was. It was a victory – we succeeded in changing the building, and there … the access was more central, more accessible also in terms of information. (Ituiutaba, Brazil)

We worked more fulfilled knowing that the user had gone satisfied from the service, feeling important and that that person had taken a decision about his/her life and health. So, that was remarkable as much professionally as in my personal life. (Campo Largo, Brazil)

I don't know if it's the most important one, as you said, but I know about the change of attitude of professionals involved, all the professionals who were involved, even those that hadn't been trained were contaminated and realized the model and tried to change something too. I think that the new attitude of professionals was the most evident result of the project. (Campo Largo, Brazil)

All the time that we start a follow-up meeting and we asked what changed, everybody said that now they attended the users in a most positive way, the user is really a subject, a person that has rights. (Vespasiano, Brazil)

Improvements in service delivery and training also faced major difficulties, among which leadership change or inadequacies in leadership stand out as important barriers. As long as the team of municipal trainers and innovators had good leadership, many of the bureaucratic and even financial constraints could be overcome and remarkable successes were achieved. When leaders and key staff changed, however – in the wake of elections or for other reasons – or when the key coordinators were simply not working effectively with the team, progress was slower and more limited. Also, issues requiring repeated action, such as ensuring regular purchases of contraceptive supplies, were difficult to sustain. A detailed discussion of the larger institutional, bureaucratic and political issues that have stood in the way of implementing change is provided in Chapter 7.

Lessons and conclusions

The experience of implementing training programmes in Brazil, Bolivia and Chile for over six years validates the importance of the three central components of Reprolatina's approach:

- anchoring a participatory and comprehensive educational process in the philosophy of Paulo Freire and the vision of the ICPD;
- combining training with the creation of an enabling environment;
- building training capacity as a central element of scaling up.

Although not a magic bullet, Reprolatina's educational process generated essential actions in participating municipalities that began to transform the way reproductive health services are conceptualized and delivered. Participants reacted with a sense of fulfilment to the training and its methodology, indicating that this type of approach is what motivates them to work to implement the ICPD agenda. Public sector health systems in Latin America lack stability as a result of political changes and health reforms that are not well understood at the local level. Reprolatina's educational process was instrumental in increasing the morale and motivation of the health team, helping it to mobilize the community and to strengthen sexual and reproductive health services.

More than six years of experience and focus group results also confirmed the value of combining formal training with a range of other interventions that enable trainers to function in their new roles and implement change. Clear understandings and agreements with local authorities about the training-led change process could not always guarantee long-term support, but it was an essential ingredient for success. Continued and empowerment-focused supervision from the Reprolatina team provided much needed support with problem solving and inspiration. The electronic communications network in turn facilitated supervision and the exchange of information with the Reprolatina team and other municipal partners.

A key component of Reprolatina's scaling-up strategy – developing local training capacity – was also validated. In most of the municipalities, local trainers succeeded in training other municipal providers and in meeting the training needs resulting from staff turnover. Some newly trained trainers were able to take on responsibility for training providers in other municipalities. The capability to train new staff ensured sustainability; whereas training of other providers in the same or another municipality brought the benefits of Reprolatina's approach to new people and new areas.

Perhaps the greatest insight to be gained from engaging in the form of participatory education as advocated by Paulo Freire and practised by Reprolatina is the realization that change is possible: the way things are is not the way they have to be. A second key lesson from Reprolatina's experience is that transformative training and associated interventions are not short-term, one-time events; they are intensive endeavours requiring long time horizons because the quantum of change implied in these innovations is very large (see Chapter 2).

It took the sustained attention of a small nongovernmental training institution six years, as well as considerable financial resources, to achieve the results reported here. Moreover, given that the amount of change implied in the training and the related innovations is large, there are inherent limitations in the number of municipalities in which Reprolatina could work. This then, is a basic lesson of the experience: the far-reaching, transformational changes called for cannot happen quickly and cannot be scaled up dramatically if the resource team is a small, nongovernmental training institution.

Reprolatina's strategy of building training capacity made a major contribution in helping to sustain and expand the innovations. Nonetheless, the impact of this newly created training capacity on scaling up is also limited. Trainers have not been able to put into practice all the planned activities because they have to divide their time between multiple tasks: training and provision of services in reproductive health and other areas of primary health care. Moreover, political-administrative relationships among municipalities in a decentralized health system do not always encourage use of trainers from one municipality to conduct training in another (see Chapter 7).

The reproductive and other health-care challenges facing developing countries require that service provision be strengthened. The approach to training and scaling up described in this paper provides a methodology for getting such a strengthening process under way. Large-scale success, however, requires more than the work of a single, small NGO. The challenge thus remains to discover how such a powerful training methodology can be transferred more widely to the public sector and incorporated into the curricula of universities and other health professional training programmes.

Acknowledgements

Very special appreciation goes to Ruth Simmons for her ongoing assistance with the conceptualization and writing of this paper. We would also like to thank the many other people who reviewed the paper and provided input: Juan Díaz, Peter Fajans, Laura Ghiron, Max Heirich, Nancy Newton, Alexis Ntabona, Jeremy Shiffman, and Maxine Whittaker. We are extremely grateful for financial support from the Bill and Melinda Gates Foundation. Finally, we could not have implemented the training programmes described in this paper without the confidence and trust the trainees and the municipalities placed in us. We are deeply grateful for their support.

References

1. *Beijing Declaration*. Fourth World Conference on Women, Beijing, September 1995 (http://www.un.org/womenwatch/daw/beijing/platform/declar.htm, accessed 21 February 2006).

2. *Programme of Action adopted at the International Conference on Population and Development, Cairo, 5–13 September 1994*. New York, United Nations Population Fund, 1996.

3. *United Nations Millennium Declaration*. New York, United Nations, 2000 (United Nations General Assembly Resolution A/55/2, 18 September 2000; http://www.un.org/millennium/declaration/ares552e.pdf, accessed 1 March 2006).

4. Simmons R, Hall P, Díaz J et al. The strategic approach to contraceptive introduction. *Studies in Family Planning*, 1997, 28:79–94.

5. *The strategic approach to improving reproductive health policies and programmes: a summary of experiences*. Geneva, World Health Organization, 2002 (Department of Reproductive Health and Research, WHO/RHR/02.12).

6. Formiga JN, Diniz SG, Simmons R et al. *An assessment of the need for contraceptive introduction in Brazil*. Geneva, World Health Organization, 1994 (Special Programme of Research, Development and Research Training in Human Reproduction, WHO/HRP/ITT/94.2).

7. Camacho HV, de la Galvez A, Paz M et al. *Diagnóstico cualitativo de la atención en salud reproductiva en Bolivia [Qualitative assessment of reproductive health services in Bolivia]*. Geneva, World Health Organization, 1996 (Special Programme of Research, Development and Research Training in Human Reproduction, WHO/HRP/ITT/96.1).

8. Díaz M, Simmons R, Díaz J et al. Expanding contraceptive choice: findings from Brazil. *Studies in Family Planning*, 1999, 30:1–16.

9. Díaz M, Simmons R, Díaz J et al. Action research to enhance reproductive choice in a Brazilian municipality: the Santa Barbara Project. In: Haberland N, Measham D, eds. *Responding to Cairo: case-studies of changing practice in reproductive health and family* planning. New York, The Population Council, 2001:355–375.

10. French WL, Bell CH. *Organization development: behavioral science interventions for organization improvement*, International 6th ed. Englewood Cliffs, NJ, Prentice-Hall, 1995.

11. Bruce J. Fundamental elements of the quality of care: a simple framework. *Studies in Family Planning*, 1990, 21:61–91.

12. Díaz M, Simmons R. When is research participatory? Reflections on a reproductive health project in Brazil. *Journal of Women's Health*, 1999, 8:175–184.

13. Penteado LG, Cabral F, Díaz M et al. Organizing a public-sector vasectomy program in Brazil. *Studies in Family Planning*, 2001, 32:315–328.

14. *Evaluating World Health Organization Project 96323: Brazil Stage III: Researching the utilization and dissemination of findings from a project on the improvement of contraceptive choice within the context of reproductive health. Final technical report*. São Paulo, Centro de Pesquisas Materno-Infantis de Campinas (CEMICAMP) [Centre for Mother and Child Research of Campinas], 2000 (unpublished).

15. Barretto V. *Paulo Freire para educadores [Paulo Freire for educators]*, 3rd ed. São Paulo, Arte e Ciência, 1998.

16. Freire P. *Pedagogia do oprimido [Pedagogy of the oppressed]*, 29th ed. São Paulo, Paz e Terra, 2000.

17. Freire P. *Pedagogia da autonomia: saberes necessários à prática educativa*.

[Pedagogy of autonomy: necessary knowledge for educational practice], 17th ed. São Paulo, Paz e Terra, 2001.

18. Pucci B. Teoria crítica e educação [Critical theory and education]. In: Pucci B, ed. *Teoria crítica e educação: a questão da formação cultural na escola de Frankfurt [Critical theory and education: the question of cultural development in the Frankfurt School]*, 2nd ed. São Paolo, Vozes; São Carlos, EDU-FISCAR, 1995:11–58.

19. Patton MQ. Developmental evaluation. *Evaluation Practice*, 1994, 15:311–319.

20. Fetterman DM. *Foundations of empowerment evaluation*. Thousand Oaks, CA, Sage Publications, 2001.

Conclusions

This book has brought together insights from a comprehensive review of relevant literature, as well as the experience of major scaling-up initiatives in family planning and primary care services from Africa, Asia and Latin America. We hope that the value of conducting systematic analysis of the determinants of successful scaling up has been demonstrated by this effort.

Most of the understanding about scaling up presented here stems from experiences with the expansion of family planning and related reproductive health services. In all of these cases, efforts were focused on improving public sector programmes. The relevance of the conceptual frameworks and the lessons that have emerged from the authors' experiences, however, extend beyond these areas of application. As Skibiak et al. argued in discussing the Zambian experience in Chapter 4, "the greatest challenges in scaling up reside in the practical, organizational transformation of a small pilot study to a broad-based programmatic intervention". The strategic choices that have to be made and the determinants of success apply across sectors and across different types of implementing agencies. Therefore the principles and lessons discussed here are not limited to reproductive health or to the public sector, but can also be of value when adapted to other areas of health and development.

Because work on this book has benefited from several opportunities for ongoing intellectual exchange over a period of years, those who participated have been able to use the lessons learned to shape scaling-up activities in the field. At the same time we wish to clarify that this is not a cookbook from which project managers can select specific, step-by-step recipes. It can, however, provide general principles and examples to be used in the development of scaling-up strategies uniquely appropriate to their context.

The same type of marriage between universal principles and the need for local relevance and adaptation applies to the innovations discussed here. New ways of improving equitable access to good health services or of implementing strategies that empower women, communities or young people to demand quality of care, for example, must be backed by locally generated evidence. Concepts and case-studies, or internationally accepted best practices, can offer guidance on what general principles are relevant, but they do not provide detailed operational plans for how quality of care and service access can be enhanced in a specific country, province or district. Such planning requires context-specific diagnostic assessments, designs and testing through pilot or experimental projects.

Throughout this volume we have defined scaling up as deliberate efforts to increase the impact of health service innovations locally tested in pilot or experimental projects, so as to benefit more people and to foster policy and programme development on a lasting basis. As was seen in the case-studies from Bangladesh and Ghana, such testing may have to be repeated. In both countries, results from experimental projects were rejected as irrelevant for national policy because innovations had been tested under special circumstances with major inputs from research institutions. They were therefore not considered to be models applicable to other parts of the country which work under more severe resource constraints. Further evidence, generated under realistic local conditions, was demanded before leaders would commit themselves to nationwide scaling up. Moreover, ongoing monitoring is needed – especially in situations of great diversity – to ensure that the innovation is producing the desired results in the process of expansion and adaptation.

Although introduction of new practices typically requires some locally generated evidence before scaling up begins, the extent of local testing needed is a function of the "quantum of change" implied by the interventions. One does not normally think of the degree of change as a variable in scaling up, but in the process of our work we have learned that it is a major factor. The innovations discussed in this book all amount to a significant degree of change in the way health service systems function, they required a package of interventions, rather than the introduction of a single new measure. Building capacity to provide informed choice, balanced information, a respect for reproductive rights, empowerment-focused training, client-centred participatory approaches or community-based services implies major change in resource-poor public sector programmes. It is important to think about the degree of change from the time that service innovations are designed and tested, through the stage when they are expanded to new areas or settings. As already noted, we must begin with the end in mind.

Because scaling up, as discussed here, is an institution-building process, it takes time. Institutions do not change overnight but require considerable nurturing to learn how to function in new ways. As an institution-building task with a focus on sustainability, scaling up requires longer time horizons than those frequently mandated by donor agencies and policy-makers keen to show results. The means and resources necessary to ensure successful and sustainable scaling up are therefore at odds with a "project" perspective which expects that results can be achieved in two or three years.

One of the key conclusions from our work is that scaling up requires support from a resource team whose members play a catalytic role, helping governments find ways to bring about change. In all of the case-studies, the expansion and institutionalization of innovations benefited from the efforts of a group of professionals – either inside or outside government, either formally designated or not – who facilitated the scaling-up process. They played major roles in advocacy, research and technical assistance with planning, strategizing, the development of training curricula and materials for information, education and communication as well as with resource mobilization. These resource teams received at least some support from external donors.

We hope that our work will lead to wide recognition that the roles played by the resource team are vital for scaling up. These functions are not the same as managing routine programme implementation. Consequently, the teams are unlikely to be funded by governments struggling to finance their weak service delivery systems. Such teams are the engine that drives change, creating public sector capacity for, and ownership of, service delivery innovations. This capacity building was demonstrated again and again in the cases discussed in this book, where individuals who had initially participated in scaling up as members of the user organization soon began to function as members of the resource team. Donor investments and ongoing support for these innovators are extremely important and are likely to have major pay-offs.

Many of the insights on scaling up presented in this volume derive from what is referred to as open-systems thinking in the organization sciences. Open-systems thinking draws attention to the interrelations between organizations and their larger sociocultural, political, economic and institutional environments. Scaling up is not exclusively a technical and managerial undertaking unaffected by the outside world. It is influenced by persistent gender inequality and other cultural factors, the extent of poverty in a country, the capacity of the national health sector and its bureaucratic institutions, historical legacies, and the nature of the political system. Scaling up in Bangladesh, for example, depended more on formal, bureaucratic organizations than in Ghana where grassroots partnerships among traditional leaders, politicians and health professionals were the driving force. These contrasts were grounded in different historical and bureaucratic traditions as well as in different patterns of social organization.

In Brazil, a highly decentralized health sector, combined with political sensitivities surrounding family planning, imposed severe limits on scaling up. At the same time, detailed knowledge of how the health sector functions under decentralization made it possible to identify and mobilize resources for expanding innovations. The importance of navigating the multiple and varied environments of scaling up and of utilizing the opportunities that arise, is one of the main lessons with which we wish to leave our readers.

Systems thinking shows that the innovation, the resource team, the user organization, the environment and the scaling-up strategy interact with each other, often in complex ways. To contend with this dynamic interplay, strategies must aim for balance or congruence among the elements of scaling up. Achieving balance is the ideal, but in reality it is neither easy nor always possible. The ideal conditions for scaling up rarely or never exist, and choices typically will have to be made within a constrained environment. Attempts to balance the relative strengths and weaknesses among the elements tend to result in compromise or trade-offs. As we saw in the case-studies, the greater the degree of change implied in the innovation, the greater will be the need for resources and support from a strong resource team and the slower will be the pace of expansion. Alternatively, if there is pressure for more rapid scaling up, or if support from the resource team is inadequate, the greater is the likelihood that the humanitarian and social equity values that are the foundation of health service innovations will be lost. When there is pressure for rapid scaling up to serve a greater number of people, as frequently occurs, the resource team needs to grow and develop its capacity.

Even the most solidly designed scaling-up strategy, which has carefully weighed all the opportunities and constraints presented by the context, will be implemented in an ever-changing environment. In Viet Nam, scaling up quality of care interventions began when the country's political system was still highly centralized, but as scaling up progressed, so did the process of health sector reform and decentralization. A strategy developed for a strongly centralized administrative system became less appropriate as decentralization took effect.

Remaining flexible and relevant in the midst of expansion emerged in these studies as a major determinant of successful scaling up. Flexibility and local autonomy to participate in decisions encourages local ownership and appropriate action on the ground. As the Zambia case-study showed, however, effective use of organizational resources at levels above the district can produce economies of scale, facilitating scaling up in ways that districts working on their own could not have accomplished. Clearly, what works best is local autonomy and ownership, coupled with strong support and initiatives at higher levels that create an enabling environment and put structures in place in which local action can flourish.

In other words, both horizontal scaling up (expansion/replication) and vertical scaling up (political, legal and institutional actions) are essential. Several of the case-studies illustrate this principle. In China, the ability to demonstrate that substantial quality-of-care improvements could be undertaken in an expanding number of counties was critical for persuading policy-makers to incorporate the principles of informed choice and voluntarism into new legislation and operational programme procedures. Alternatively, the Community-based Health Planning and Services initiative in Ghana, which was driven largely by peer exchanges among districts, could not progress without national-level support in the form of training and human resource development. In Brazil, expansion of training innovations was constrained because opportunities for vertical scaling up were limited.

It is not unusual for researchers and professionals to close with a plea for more research. We are no exception, basing our argument on two key points. First, research should not be limited to the testing of the innovation. Rather, continued research should guide the process of scaling up, providing ongoing input into strategy design and adaptations, as well as providing information that allows appropriate monitoring. Second, as we hope this book has demonstrated, research facilitates understanding of the determinants of successful scaling up and identifies the type of financial and technical support needed. Moreover, as innovations are adapted to local contexts, there may come a point where the evidence base for the success of the original innovative service package is no longer relevant. Continued monitoring and research should examine whether the benefits of the innovation continue to be present in the process of adaptation and expansion. In the most general sense, research builds international and local understanding of how to expand small-scale health service innovations so as to benefit more people, more quickly, more lastingly.

Much remains to be learned about scaling up, and this book is by no means the final word on the subject. We hope, however, that the materials presented here will stimulate new ideas and insights among researchers and practitioners that will lead to much needed improvements in sexual and reproductive health services. Given that scaling up is in essence a managerial, organizational and political task, the perspectives and conclusions from our work should also be useful for a wider array of health and development efforts.